# Suicide and the Self



This book centres on self-accounts of suicidal behaviour, using a Critical Discourse Analysis (CDA) approach to offer a qualitative perspective within current suicidology and suicide prevention research.

*Suicide and the Self: A Discourse Analysis Approach to Self-Narratives of Suicide* is the first qualitative study to explore suicide through the eyes of the person experiencing it. The volume is grounded in foundational CDA concepts, which view social reality as constructed through language and draw on data from real people's writings, interviews, visual representations, and farewell letters to understand the discursive resources and linguistic patterns in these narratives from varied temporal perspectives.

By focusing on how individuals construct their own stories, Galasiński and Ziółkowska show how a discourse analytic approach can enrich suicidological research and inform suicide prevention efforts. This book is essential reading for scholars in suicidology, medical humanities, allied health, and discourse analysis.

**Dariusz Galasiński** is a Professor in the Institute of Journalism at the University of Wroclaw, Poland.

**Justyna Ziółkowska** is an Associate Professor at the Department of Clinical Psychology, SWPS University, Poland.

## Routledge Research in Language and Communication

**The Discursive Construction of Place in the Digital Age**
*Edited by Alejandro Parini and Francisco Yus*

**Perspectives on Knowledge Communications**
Concepts and Settings
*Edited by Jan Engberg, Antoinette Fage-Butler, and Peter Kastberg*

**Multidisciplinary Approaches to the Discourses of Extremism**
*Edited by Katie Jane Patterson and Encarnación Hidalgo-Tenorio*

**Multidisciplinary Views on Discourse Genre**
A Research Agenda
*Edited by Ninke Stukker, John A. Bateman, Danielle McNamara, and Wilbert Spooren*

**Talking Images**
The Interface between Drawing and Writing
*Edited by Silvia Ferrara, Mattia Cartolano, and Ludovica Ottaviano*

**Semioethics as Existential Dialogue**
The Gift and Burden of Responsibility
*Edited by Susan Petrilli and Susan Mancino*

**Framing Sustainability in Language and Communication**
*Edited by Maida Kosatica and Sean P. Smith*

**Suicide and the Self**
A Discourse Analysis Approach to Self-Narratives of Suicide
*Dariusz Galasiński and Justyna Ziółkowska*

For more information about this series, please visit: www.routledge.com/Routledge-Research-in-Language-and-Communication/book-series/RRLC

# Suicide and the Self

## A Discourse Analysis Approach to Self-Narratives of Suicide

**Dariusz Galasiński and Justyna Ziółkowska**

Routledge
Taylor & Francis Group
NEW YORK AND LONDON

First published 2025
by Routledge
605 Third Avenue, New York, NY 10158

and by Routledge
4 Park Square, Milton Park, Abingdon, Oxon, OX14 4RN

*Routledge is an imprint of the Taylor & Francis Group, an informa business*



ISBN: 9781032672823 (hbk)
ISBN: 9781032672861 (pbk)
ISBN: 9781032672847 (ebk)

DOI: 10.4324/9781032672847

Typeset in Sabon
by Newgen Publishing UK

# Contents

1 Suicide and the Self 1

2 Self in Suicide 38

3 Self and Agency 63

4 Romanticisation of Suicide 86

5 Self in Interaction 109

6 Parents and Suicide 128

7 Legacy of the Self 151

8 The Emotional Self 172

9 Conclusions 198

*Index* *212*

# 1 Suicide and the Self

## Introduction

This book is about stories of people who either took or attempted to take their lives. It is about the individual perspective on suicide, as told in accounts of those engaged in suicidal behaviour. Who do they say they are? What are they like? What did they do when doing suicide? How did they imagine themselves after the act? We pose these and other questions having studied suicide letters of people who took their lives and interviews of those who survived their suicide attempts.

'Each suicide drama occurs in the mind of a unique individual' (Shneidman, 1996, p. 5). Shneidman's famous words about suicide reflect well the perspective on suicide we want to take in this book. In contrast to the dominant suicidological view, we aim to focus on the individual experiences of people who decided to take the step of taking their lives. We want to understand suicide and its processes as socially situated, which, in contrast to what Shneidman proposes, do not only happen in a person's mind but also in particular social contexts through which suicide is made sense by both the person who ends their life and those who stay behind and must understand what happened.

The book is founded on our continued surprise that individual suffering, decisions, and tragedies continue to be represented as part of global statistics on suicide. In contrast, we want to see the person who wishes to or eventually takes their life through their eyes. This book looks at stories of suicide as performed by persons in particular situations. The aim is to understand how people who engaged in the process of taking their own life described themselves and those around them. We also focus on those people as they are narrated in their stories.

We also stress the importance of discourse analysis in suicidology and suicide prevention. We argue that studying narratives on suicide and the reality they represent adds significantly to understanding suicide,

DOI: 10.4324/9781032672847-1

particularly its experiences and meanings. Discourse analytic insights enrich and contextualise the existing suicidological knowledge.

The macro-level view of suicide dominates in suicidology as individuals become parts of social groups at different levels of generality. Suicide and suicide attempts have rarely been seen as 'private' events. They are usually studied as points on a timeline, while their contexts are seen in terms of a multitude of correlations. Suicides have also rarely been studied as involving 'real people' but rather as sets of demographics necessary for statistical calculations. Suicide is not seen as a process in which people are involved in a variety of actions, some of which result in their death, an act that is underpinned by multiple stories of the person, their views, emotions, or expectations.

We want to reverse the top-down perspective and start with an individual's experience as it is related in their story. It is these experiences that are central to our discussion here. Reversing the top-down perspective and focusing firmly on narrated experiences allows us to obtain new insights on suicide and contextualise the existing knowledge about it. Indeed, despite repeated and frequent calls from suicidology for a significant increase in qualitative bottom-up research (e.g., Hjelmeland & Knizek, 2010; Bantjes & Swartz, 2019), its application in studies on suicide and/or suicide attempts remains obscure. At the same time, research into the context-situated person involved in suicide and/or suicide attempts is practically non-existent.

## Aims of the Book

The overall aim of the book is to shed light on the perspective of the individual in how suicide and its process are narrated. Our aim is to examine discursively constructed subjectivities of people who either took their own lives or made a serious attempt to do so. How did they construct themselves in their own stories? Who did they speak as?

We are interested in two main themes in stories of suicide. First, we focus on the individual. How do they position themselves and their actions with regard to the act? How do they position the act itself and its aftermath? In particular, we explore issues of agency in suicide—we want to see where it is primarily located, and how it is constructed. Second, we are interested in how stories of suicide construct relationships with the person who is about to or wants to take their life. How do they see their legacy? How do they see their emotionality? In a nutshell, this book is about the narrated experience of an individual either facing suicide or telling the story after they survived. We want to shed light on what it means to experience suicide as an individual in a social context.

As we explore discourses from and about people who were probably at the most dramatic juncture of their lives, we are also interested in their form. With what certainty do people telling their suicide stories speak? What acts of communication are they engaged in? How do they position themselves in terms of control and agency?

As suicidology considers gender a key dimension in understanding suicide, we are interested in the extent and contexts to which gendered positions are accessed (or oriented to) in the texts we analyse. In other words, to what extent do people who are about to end their lives or make a serious attempt on their life speak as men or women? We locate their experience within the society's ways of constructing gender.

Our book has another aim. We believe that combining two sets of data—interviews with individuals with experience of a suicide attempt and suicide notes—is the most fruitful way to gain insight into suicide experience. Yet, suicidology is barely interested in individual experiences, and it is even less interested in suicide notes. In contrast, we believe individual stories, whether spoken or rendered in suicide notes, offer the most interesting and ecological insight into the process of suicide.

So, by combining a corpus of interviews and suicide notes, we want to show that the two corpora offer complementary insights and should probably be analysed next to each other. As we suggest increased effort towards qualitative suicidology, we want to stress the usefulness of combining what has so far been two separate areas of research. Our work is an effort to promote text-based suicidological research as one area of study.

## The Book's Projects

Similar to our previous book (Galasiński & Ziółkowska, 2020), this book rises out of our continued frustration with the dominant discourses of suicidology. Time and again, we see suicide constructed as a single and largely uncomplicated event that can be explained by a set of risk factors. We want to challenge this assumed simplicity of suicide. Suicide does not just happen; it consists of a set of activities that are constitutive of it.

Therefore, contrary to the dominant suicidological views, we seek to show the drama of suicide. We aim to show that at the centre of suicide, there is an individual with a unique perspective on themselves and those around them. Moreover, the individual is engaged in a process that extends well beyond applying lethal action to oneself. This is why the first project of the book is to continue bringing attention to the complexity of suicide.

This book is about the most dramatic event of anyone's life; it is about people's suffering. The stories we heard in interviews and read in suicide notes were heart-wrenching. They were stories of rejection and self-rejection, failure, and concealment, topped with unconditional love and yearning for reciprocity, which in most cases, never came. We were in touch with raw human misery. As we delve into their suffering, we want to write about them as more than a contribution to another statistical calculation or model. We are interested in the stories of people at life's edge. We hope that this book will do them justice.

We also understand that our book is largely polemical, and our third project is to offer an alternative view on suicide and suicide prevention. We believe that increasingly accepted qualitative perspectives in suicidology offer important contributions to understanding and preventing suicide. By understanding experiences of suicide, we begin to understand its social meanings; through this, we begin to understand better how to design prevention and clinical interventions. We are interested in setting up a dialogue between qualitative discourse analysis and the mainstream discourses of suicide, both in suicidology and in suicide prevention.

## Suicide

Deaths by suicide are high. Every 40 seconds, someone in the world takes their life, making up almost a million individuals a year (World Health Organization [WHO], 2024). Hudzik and Cannon (2014) report that more people die in suicidal acts than in wars or murders. According to the Eurostat, the 2021 suicide rate in the European Union (EU) was 10.2 suicides per 100,000 people. The lowest (2.7/100,100) was in Cyprus, while the highest was in Slovenia (19.8/100,000) (Eurostat, 2024). There are, of course, even more suicide attempts. Cautious estimates indicate that the number of suicide attempts is 10–15 times greater than the number of suicides. However, the American Foundation for Suicide Prevention (AFSP) estimates that 0.6% of adults aged 18 or older made at least one suicide attempt (American Foundation for Suicide Prevention [AFSP], 2024).

Men commit considerably more suicides than women; it is considerably more in high-income countries. This is the essence of the so-called gender paradox in suicide. Canetto and Sakinofsky (1998) observe that while women have a higher incidence of suicide ideation and behaviour, more men take their lives. The numbers are quite worrying. Men's suicide rates have been increasing in the twentieth century (Canetto, 2017; also Pitman et al., 2012; River & Flood, 2021, Oliffe et al., 2018). In 2016, the global male–female suicide ratio was 1.8, whereas it was significantly higher in some European countries. In our native Poland, the male–female suicide ratio goes beyond 7:1, while in Lithuania, it is just under 7 (WHO, 2019). More men take their lives in almost all countries in the world than women; according to the WHO in 2016, there were only seven countries (from 183 listed) where women took their lives more than men.

Over the centuries, attitudes towards suicide have changed significantly. In ancient Greece, suicide was accepted, especially if it was done for an important reason (e.g., bereavement, illness, or honour [O'Connor & Sheehy, 2000]). This tolerant attitude started changing with the rise of Christianity and the commandment not to kill under whose purview suicide fell. Suicide became an act against the 'natural law' (Hecht, 2013). Consequently, a person who committed suicide became a perpetrator of a crime (Minois, 2001; Marsh, 2013).

The beginning of the nineteenth century brought a new perspective on suicide. It was the first time suicide was perceived either as an illness or a symptom of an illness (Marsh, 2010; Hacking, 1990). Doctors received powers to secure, treat, control, and assess suicide (Hacking, 1990). Nowadays, the common assumption is that suicide is a result of mental health problems (Battin, 1995; Pridmore, 2011; Marsh, 2010). A person who takes their life is represented as someone who suffers psychologically and kills themselves when they are in a bad psychological state. Common are publications in which authors state that one cannot commit suicide unless they are mentally ill (e.g., Mościcki, 1997; Harris & Barraclough, 1997). A medicalised view of suicide is adopted beyond psychiatry; it is, for example, adopted by the United Nations' World Health Organization (WHO).

Indeed, the medical view of suicide was recently strengthened. In the *Diagnostic and Statistical Manual of Mental Disorders, Fifth Edition (DSM-V)*, the American Psychiatric Association (APA) indicated that it would look into suicidal behaviour to determine whether it should be treated as a mental disorder called Suicidal Behaviour Disorder (APA, 2013; 2022). This is underscored by claims that suicide ideation can now be reduced pharmacologically (Huang et al., 2022).

As might be expected, further medicalisation of suicide is controversial (for a review of objections to a suicidality-specific diagnosis, see Obegi, 2019). Some argue that taking suicidal behaviour as a separate disorder will allow the development of uniform terminology and improve the quality of research (see Oliogu & Ruocco, 2024; Fehling & Selby, 2021). Moreover, it is argued that such a move would enhance suicide prevention. Indeed, WHO estimates that as many as 165,000 people could be protected from suicide annually if they received adequate psychiatric help (Bertolote et al., 2003).

However, the counter-argument is that medicine can hardly deal with suicidal behaviour it knows little about. People take their lives despite psychiatric help and medication (Maris, 2015; Hengartner et al., 2021). Arguments that suicide results from a mental disorder are countered with research that there are suicides where no mental illness was ever determined (e.g., Schmutte et al., 2021; Milner, Sveticic, & De Leo, 2013; Phillips, 2010).

Furthermore, suicide prevention is largely based on the biomedical model of suicide. Despite many efforts, suicide rates tend to stay the same, while predicting suicide remains in the realm of fanciful aspiration (Pokorny, 1983; 1993; Belsher et al., 2019). Indeed, it is the social understanding that seems to offer more promising perspectives on suicide and its prevention. There are more suicides in deprived communities than in their non-deprived counterparts (Cairns, Graham, & Bambra, 2017). Such research builds on earlier studies that suggest that unemployment (up to four times) and other economic factors such as indebtedness significantly increase the risk of suicide (Mäki & Martikainen, 2012; Sinyor et al., 2024). The medicalisation of suicide will hardly help here.

Finally, despite many terminologies and classification systems, so far none has been adopted universally. It is clear, however, that an ideal system should be atheoretical and acultural, and consist of mutually exclusive concepts that comprise the full spectrum of suicidal behaviours and ideation (Silverman & De Leo, 2016). Although doubts are expressed as to the possibility of arriving at such a classification, the goal remains an important one (Goodfellow, Kõlves, & De Leo, 2019).

### *Suicide and Suicide Attempt*

An act of suicide is when one's actions lead to an intended outcome, death; the person is aware of what their actions will lead to (De Leo et al., 2006; Klonsky, May, & Saffer, 2016). A suicide attempt, on the other hand, is an act of suicide in which death did not occur (Posner et al., 2007; Crosby, Ortega, & Melanson, 2011). The crucial aspect of a suicide attempt is the existence of suicidal intent, that is to say, the intention to take one's own life. In both cases, the requirement of the intent to end one's own life in the definition of suicidal action raises difficult issues of determining such an intention after someone's death or even after an attempt.

Although the term 'suicide attempt' is used widely and without rigour that it might mean nothing (O'Carroll et al., 1996), both clinical and research interests in it remain high. The suicide attempt is the most important predictor of suicide (Franklin et al., 2017; Riera-Serra et al., 2024). This fact alone suggests the significance of research into suicide attempts, as it is such experiences that give significant insight into suicide and its process.

We realise that some researchers question the status of homogeneous suicide attempts. Meehan, Lamb, Saltzman, and O'Carroll (1992) demonstrated that only one in ten suicide attempts resulted in hospitalisation; only another two required medical attention while the lethality of the remaining 70% is unknown. Other research shows that more than half of the people who attempt suicide do not seek medical help (Crosby, Cheltenham,

& Sacks, 1999). It is reasonable to ask, therefore, whether suicide attempts resulting in such drastically different consequences are a group of similar events. Unfortunately, although there are postulates that suicide attempts should also be assessed for their lethality (Williams, 2014), there is still no universal method of doing it. Interestingly, when asked to assess 10 cases of possible suicide attempts, 14 suicidologists and 59 clinicians could not agree on much, even though half of the participants were provided with a definition of the suicide attempt (Wagner et al., 2002). To a considerable extent, therefore, a suicide attempt is something that is socially constructed between the person who attempts to takes their life, possibly their family, and the clinician who acknowledges it and admits the person for care.

## Suicide and the Self

Suicide is always about the self. It is always an act of an individual in their unique social, cultural, and psychological contexts. This is reflected in definitions of suicide as well as in suicide theories, which put the individual at the centre of the act of suicide. So, sometimes an individual is helpless in their psychache, which is caused by deprivation of vital needs; they cannot see another way out besides suicide (Shneidman, 1996). It may be an individual who sees suicide as an escape from the suicidal self and its suffering (Baumeister, 1990). Joiner (2005), alternatively, proposes to see the self as experiencing thwarted belongingness, which, together with the feeling of being a burden, creates motivation for suicide. Van Orden, Witte, Cukrowicz, Braithwaite, Selby, and Joiner (2010) also add resulting feelings of hopelessness as a motivator. There are also feelings of helplessness, defeat, or entrapment (O'Connor, 2011; Williams, 1997).

In all conceptual accounts of suicide known to us, the individual who experiences themselves in the world surrounding them is at the centre of how suicide is understood. And yet, despite the centrality of individual experience in suicide, the individual vanishes in suicidological research. This happens both in suicidology and, for example, in sociological accounts of suicide that are explicitly interested in looking at suicide in terms of its social context (see Durkheim, 1897/1966; Johnson, 1965; Henry & Short, 1954). It is tenable to say that, by and large, researchers are uninterested in the individual they place at the centre of understanding suicide.

Research on suicide focuses on two levels. On the one hand, it is social groups, offering insight at the levels of demography and/or epidemiology. On the other, researchers examine specific variables, isolated aspects of the human psyche, which are postulated to be associated with suicidal behaviour. For example, there is research into relationships between perfectionism and suicide (Smith et al., 2018), shame and guilt in self-harm (Sheehy et al., 2019), or resiliency and its role in suicidal behaviour

(Shahram et al., 2021). What is common in such vast research is ignoring the individual experience of a person and focusing on its aspect, which is turned into a theory-driven abstract construct representing, sometimes, a minute aspect of human experience away from the context in which it occurs.

By far most of such research is done within the positivist, quantitative paradigm, based on the hypothetical-deductive model that requires rejecting the complexity of the studied phenomena. Such research focuses on selected aspects that are positioned as objects that can be manipulated and measured. In such a way, what constitutes complex human experience in a particular context is removed from the researcher's sight (Gergen, 1973; Harré, 1979). The self in suicide vanishes.

In contrast to the dominant paradigm, this book is primarily interested in the individual experience as it is narrated by the individual. We want to explore how the individual narrates themselves with regard to the suicidal actions they undertake. In exploring such experiences, we are particularly interested in how people engaged in suicidal action construct themselves in terms of their agency. In other words, as suicide is consistently conceptualised in terms of individual agency, we are therefore interested in how such agency is constructed in stories of lived experiences of suicide.

It also means we are interested in how writers of suicide notes and interviewees position themselves as doing things in their suicidal actions. We want to examine who is positioned as doing which kind of things in relation to what or whom. To do this, we focus on the lexicogrammatical form of the texts we analyse, rather than on their contents.

### *Agency in Suicide*

Agency is an individual's capacity to act intentionally and put this capacity into action. Such an understanding of agency is a key dimension of suicide, which is consistently understood as the foundation of the suicidal act (our review of definitions of suicide can be found in Chapter 2). Münster and Broz (2016) argue that although suicide is a volitional and agentive act, its agency is partly denied. Depression, gender, genetics, sexual orientation, or financial crises are all invoked as causes of suicide beyond the individual's control. The two researchers describe such denials as the dialectic of agency and patiency. They suggest simultaneous reliance on and denial of agency; they also argue that such a tension is inscribed in most vernacular discourses about suicide, including medical, psychological, and sociological, suicidology.

When we look at the dominant theoretical models and theories in suicidology, agency of a suicidal person is rarely addressed explicitly. Agency seems to be minimised rather than stressed in suicidal action. For example, in Shneidman's model, suicide is seen as an intentional act driven by a desire to cease psychological pain. Although the individual retains agency as they actively choose suicide as a solution to their suffering, their agency is also constrained by the overwhelming nature of their pain, which limits their ability to see other options. Consequently, while the individual makes a deliberate decision to end their life, they feel that their sense of agency is narrowed to a single option, namely that of suicide, as a result of the depth of their despair.

Suicide can be viewed as the ultimate loss of agency, a desperate act taken when individuals feel they have no other options available to them. Benson, Gibson, Boden, and Owen (2016) analysed 124 online questionnaires about the experience of suicidal feelings and 21 interviews that further explored the questionnaire data in the interview phase. They describe the suicidal self as one whose agency is disrupted and depleted. They see the experience of suicidal feelings as in opposition to agency, control, and well-being. For example, a suicidal person may experience a loss of coherence in their sense of self. As a result, the experience of self-authority of actions is threatened or even absent. A physical distance between the self and the world may also be experienced by a suicidal person. In their study, participants used metaphors such as 'bubble', 'glass wall', 'glass box', or 'coffin' to describe their experiences.

Other scholars argue for a more complex picture of agency. In their recent article discussing the state of research on the interpersonal theory of suicide, Robinson, Udupa, Rice, Wilson-Lemoine, Joiner, and Rogers (2024) link agency to the construct of hopelessness regarding belongingness and burdensomeness. They theorise that suicidal people are predominantly hopeless about their current state of perceived burdensomeness and thwarted belonging. They also believe that such states will never improve. Such a sense of helplessness, according to the researchers, constitutes a loss of agency. They argue that the suicidal person's negative experiences cannot be altered. Such a deterioration of agency in intrapersonal terms coincides with the absence of agency in interpersonal relationships. Yet, researchers argue that agency and familiarity with death (i.e., capability) increase (Robinson et al., 2024).

An equally complex picture of agency in suicide is described in ethnographic research by Imberton (2012). This is a study of how the Chol Maya indigenous people in southern Mexico attribute responsibility for suicide, and whether their understanding of agency changed as a result of social changes in the region. Imberton argues that two different logics of agency emerge from the data. On the one hand, suicide is seen as a personal and conscious choice made to escape everyday struggles. On the other, alternative explanations absolve the individual of responsibility, attributing the act to external factors such as witchcraft, drug abuse, or divine fate. These findings suggest a dual understanding of agency: one that acknowledges the victim's autonomy in choosing suicide, and another that denies this autonomy by framing the act as involuntary. Both logics coexist within local narratives, reflecting different perspectives on human agency in the context of suicide (Imberton, 2012).

In addition to being an individual trait, agency may also be shaped by broader social conditions that either facilitate or inhibit the individual's ability to cope. Some studies show the importance of environment in fostering autonomy, enhancing competence, and in the process, leading to improved mental health outcomes and a reduction in the risk of suicide. This is particularly relevant in populations that experience minority stress, such as the lesbian, gay, bisexual, transgender, and queer/questioning plus (LGBTQ+) youth, where the fulfilment of psychological needs is often compromised (Baams, Grossman, & Russell, 2015). By addressing these needs through supportive interventions, mental health professionals can potentially reduce the incidence of suicidal behaviours in vulnerable populations.

Overall, the picture of agency in suicide is ambivalent. Yet, although researchers offer mixed accounts, the conceptual models are more focused. Interestingly, critiques of the dominant models of suicide charge them with placing suicide only within the individual, while ignoring that the individual is in a social, economic, or political context that contributes to the decision. All this places agency as the key to understanding suicide. By exploring it in the narratives of lived experiences of suicide, we are interested in offering a perspective that has so far been ignored. Fitzpatrick (2016) argues that such a perspective is important also from an ethical point of view. It is crucial to recognise the agency of suicidal people and listen to their narratives to promote a nuanced understanding of their experiences (Fitzpatrick, 2016). Thus, we are interested in agency as it is lived. As far as we have been able to find out, ours is the first such account to address a significant gap in research.

### *History of Agency in Understanding Suicide*

Meanings given to agency in suicides have changed throughout history. Nowadays, agency is regarded as a core element in the perception of suicide as a bad death. In ancient Greece, attitudes to suicide were relatively tolerant. In many cases, suicide was accepted, especially if it was carried out because of bereavement, illness, or to avoid tarnishing honour (O'Connor & Sheehy, 2000). Ancient Romans had a similar attitude towards suicidal people similar to the Greeks; if it was deemed justified, it was neither judged nor condemned. Hołówka (2001) points out that suicide allowed one not to endure disgrace after a military defeat; it was proof of loyalty and allowed one to avoid punishment. However, even in these extremely tolerant times, suicide by slaves, soldiers, or people accused of crimes was forbidden and severely punished (Minois, 2001).

Tolerant attitudes towards suicide began to change in about the fifth century when the suicide victim began to be treated as the perpetrator rather than the victim (Minois, 2001; Marsh, 2013) and was therefore punished. Not only was burial denied, but the body of the suicided person was often desecrated. Burning the bodies of people who took their lives, dragging their naked bodies through the streets, dismembering and displaying them in public, piercing the bodies with a pole, burying them at a crossroads to make it difficult for their souls to orient themselves, or burying them in barrels and lowering them into a river or in the woods with other criminals were not uncommon acts (Minois, 2001). As Minois (2001) points out, the desecration of corpses persisted in Europe for a relatively long time; the most recent reports of such practices come from 1749 in Paris and 1823 in London.

The beginning of change towards such treatment of people committing suicide dates from the fourteenth to the seventeenth century. In his *Anatomy of Melancholy*, Robert Burton linked suicide to mental illness for the first time. Tondo (2014) writes that Burton placed suicide in a modern, non-religious perspective by pointing to anxiety, feelings of hopelessness, and impulsivity as factors that can influence suicidal behaviour. Undoubtedly, Burton was ahead of his time; nevertheless, from the fifteenth century onwards, other texts questioning condemnation of suicide began to appear (Hecht, 2013). Philosophers, including Montesquieu, Voltaire, Rousseau, and Hume, played their part by appealing to the idea of human freedom and stood up for the right to suicide.

Marsh (2010) argues that between the mid-seventeenth century and late eighteenth, a gradual secularisation of suicide could be observed. Suicide ceased to be explained by supernatural phenomena; instead, views appealing to rational choice and medical arguments emerged. Increasingly, suicide was seen as a result of not being in one's right mind (Latin: *non compos mentis*) rather than a crime against oneself (Latin: *felo de se*) (March, 2010). According to Williams (2014), in mid-seventeenth century England fewer than 7% of suicides were explained by the Court of King's Bench as having been committed by a person not in his right mind; by 1690, 30% of suicides were so qualified and rates gradually increased. Finally, by the end of the eighteenth century, *non compos mentis* had become the typical verdict given by the court (MacDonald, 1989).

It is worth stressing, however, that MacDonald (1989) argues that the verdict of *non compos mentis* reflected more of a social desire to spare the family of the suicide victim from the legal and theological consequences of judging suicide as a crime against oneself, rather than being an acceptance of new ideas about suicide.

A new perspective on suicide did not emerge until the beginning of the nineteenth century. The 1821 definition of suicide from the *Dictionnaire des Sciences Medicales* (Dictionary of Medical Sciences) by Jean-Etienne Esquirol is considered to be one of the landmark texts in the adoption of a medical understanding of suicide (Marsh, 2010; Hacking, 1990). Based on more than a hundred clinical cases, Esquirol defined suicide as a disease or a symptom of a disease; an internal pathology associated with excessive passion, organic changes, and classified forms of insanity. Hacking (1990) suggests that he empowered physicians to safeguard, treat, control, and evaluate suicide.

Views on suicide changed but, as argued by Marsh (2010), it is possible to distinguish three main ways in which suicide was understood in nineteenth-century publications. Initially, suicide was treated as an act resulting from anatomical pathology of the body; by the mid-nineteenth century, the source of suicide was seen as an inner impulse that overcame the individual and led to the attempt. Finally, by the end of the century, suicide was seen as a symptom of degeneration resulting from constitutional weakness.

The development of medical knowledge concerning suicide meant that suicide was gradually no longer treated as a legal problem. Legal sanctions for suicide were gradually abolished. The earliest to do so was Prussia in 1751. From then on, suicide victims were buried in a cemetery and any penalties were dropped for those who made an unsuccessful suicide attempt. In France, sanctions were abolished in 1791, 1850 in Austria, 1903 in Russia, 1931 in Italy, and as late as 1961 in England. Suicide ceased to be a punishable act in Canada and the United States of America much later.

Battin (1995) highlights that the prevailing belief is that mental problems are a factor in suicide (Pridmore, 2011; Marsh, 2010). The suicidal person is often portrayed as someone who is mentally distressed and performs the suicidal act while in a poor mental state. However, adopting a medicalised understanding of suicide does not only apply to psychiatry. Media and governmental and non-governmental agencies also link suicide to mental health problems. Examples include texts from the WHO, suicidological global organisations (www.iasp.info; www.suicidology.org) or non-governmental organisations (www.befrienders.org) that adopt the psychiatric understanding of suicidal behaviour. The need for medical care for people at risk of suicide is also enshrined in the legislation of many countries. In Poland, the *Act on Mental Health Care* mandates admission to the hospital of a person whose behaviour indicates an imminent threat to their life or the life or health of others.

De Leo (2011) draws attention to the nature of suicidal behaviour and the consequences of medicalising suicide without considering the motivation behind suicidal behaviour. He argues that assigning a psychiatric diagnosis to those who engage in suicidal behaviour is a step backwards from the contemporary multidisciplinary approach to suicide. Suicidal behaviour depends on several internal and external factors, including culture, law, and economics, and, as such, is far beyond the possibilities of medical explanation. For these reasons, treating suicidal behaviour as a disorder may do more harm than good. The categorisation of suicidal behaviour as a psychiatric disorder may also be a way to marginalise researchers who adopt other perspectives in their research; treating suicide as a multidisciplinary phenomenon will conflict with the official categorisation of suicidal acts. Needless to say, the current psychiatric thinking is in opposition to De Leo's ideas. As we discuss in the next chapter, suicide is now thoroughly medicalised as the APA is preparing to make suicidal behaviour a diagnostic entity in its own right.

In this book, we focus on agency as a characteristic of representation. We set aside the issue of the extent to which people engaged in suicidal behaviour 'really' do things or not. Rather, we seek to explore how they speak about it. How do they choose to arrange the world surrounding them and themselves in it in their narratives? To do this, we employ a version of Critical Discourse Studies, a programme of understanding discourse founded on a constructionist view of representation.

## Critical Discourse Analysis

This book is about how people communicate and the discursive resources they avail themselves of. We are interested in how suicidal action and the persons within it are narrated by those who either committed suicide or attempted to do so. We assume that such accounts give us insight into a host of meanings that allow us to understand suicide as a situated social situation experienced and given meaning by a person who performs it.

We are going to offer a brief account of a model of discourse analysis with which we have sympathy (for a much more comprehensive discussion, see Barker & Galasiński, 2001; for other such accounts, see Galasiński, 2004; 2008; 2013). In particular, the review we offer here is based on our latest ones (Galasiński & Ziółkowska, 2020; Galasiński, 2017; Ziółkowska, 2016).

We situate our analyses in a constructionist approach to discourse, and within its critical strand (Krzyżanowski & Forchtner, 2016). Thus, we draw upon a tradition in discourse analysis that is an amalgamation of several approaches including critical linguistics (Fowler et al., 1979; Hodge & Kress, 1993; Fowler, 1991), social semiotics (Hodge & Kress, 1988; Kress & van Leeuwen, 1996), sociocultural change and change in discourse (Fairclough, 1989; 1992; 1995; 2003) and socio-cognitive studies (e.g., van Dijk, 1993; 1998). Linguistically, it is anchored within systemic-functional linguistics (e.g., Halliday, 1994; 1978; Halliday & Hasan, 1985), which complements the analyst's self-reflexivity (Wodak, 1999) and can help reduce the arbitrariness of interpretation by anchoring it in the linguistic form itself.

By saying that our discourse analysis is critical, we mean that our research tackles important problems of social life and traditional issues concerning social inequalities. Indeed, we use the word 'discourse' to separate the more abstract semiotic system—language and focus on the context-bound social practice of communication—discourse.

Discourse is a form of social practice (Fowler et al., 1979) and there is a dialectic relationship between discourse and social structure. On the one hand, discourse is shaped and limited by social structures such as social class, social norms or practices; on the other hand, it is also constitutive of those structures. And so, discourse is not only a set of practices representing extralinguistic reality but also one of constructing it. It is as much the space for representation as it is for action. In such a way, every language use reproduces and, potentially, transforms the society that produced it.

We take a text-oriented approach (Fairclough, 1992). Thus, we focus on the content and the form of stretches of discourse, with an interest both in the semantics and syntax of an utterance, as well as the functions of what is said or written within the local context, and the social actions thus accomplished. Language users are engaged in communicative activities as members of social groups, organisations, institutions, and cultures. To a considerable extent, they speak the way one speaks or write as one writes—the way it is appropriate (in many senses of this word) to speak or write.

Taking a text-oriented perspective means that we separate the analytic and interpretative stages in understanding the data we approach. This is to say that the initial and main approach to the data is focused on the linguistic form of the texts, which is 'objectively' accessible. The stage of analysis will be focused on choices and patterns in vocabulary, grammar, and text structures. Such an analysis can be supported by a hermeneutic-like interpretation of discourses in terms of the context in which they were submerged (see Titscher et al., 2000). Interpretation comes after such analyses and consists of 'making sense' of the data. This process is inevitably made from the point of view of the researcher who is involved in the process. In other words, while the analysis of the linguistic form can be accepted intersubjectively, the interpretation is underpinned by individual opinion and cannot be seen as better or superior to that done from another point of view.

We are interested in the discourses (practices of representation) the interviewees and authors drew on when they spoke to us or wrote their notes. We want to discover the discourses in which the individual at the centre of the suicidal process is made social through the process of narrating themselves.

However, we are not trying to make claims as to the extent the research is representative either of how people with the experience of suicide attempt to speak or authors of suicide notes write. Rather, we are interested in uncovering the discourses underpinning their narratives to shed light on it. We are interested in uncovering the practices that construct the suicide process. Even though we cannot answer the question of how dominant these practices of representation are, the data we have, however, must be seen as informing the social context in which they are rooted.

The following assumptions we make about discourse are relevant here.

1. Discourse is socially constitutive. It is in a 'dialectical' relationship with its contexts. It as much depends on its context, as it also creates social and political 'realities' (Fairclough & Wodak, 1997; van Leeuwen & Wodak, 1999). From the notorious case of homosexuality as a former mental disease (Kutchins & Kirk, 1999) to the newly written mental illnesses such as restless legs syndrome or the so-called PMT, one can quite easily see how psychiatry invokes new diseases that psychiatrists will now treat, as people get ill from them.

   Moreover, Marsh (2010) offers a fascinating account of changes in discourses of suicide, from a personal choice, through criminalisation, all the way to its medicalisation—suicide is a symptom of mental illness and soon to become an illness in its own right.
2. Discourse is a system of options from which language users make their choices. Whatever can be said or written, can be said or written differently. Any representation of 'reality' necessarily entails decisions as to which aspects of that reality to include and how to arrange them. Each selection carries its share of socially ingrained values so that representation is socially constructed (Hall, 1997; Hodge & Kress, 1993) and alternative representations carry different significances and consequences (Fowler, 1996). Texts seek to impose a 'preferred reading' (Hall, 1981) or a 'structure of faith' (Menz, 1989) upon the addressee.
3. Discourse is ideological. The selective character of representation leads to the view that it is through discourse and other semiotic practices that ideologies are formulated, reproduced, and reinforced. We understand the term ideology as social (general and abstract) representations shared by members of a group and used by them to accomplish everyday social practices: acting and communicating (van Dijk, 1998; Billig et al., 1988; Fowler, 1985). These representations are organised into systems that are deployed by social classes and other groups 'to make sense of, figure out, and render intelligible the way society works' (Hall,

1996, p. 26), while at the same time, they are capable of 'ironing out' the contradictions, dilemmas, and antagonisms of practices in ways that accord with the interests and projects of power (Chouliaraki & Fairclough, 1999). Ideology provides us with ways in which we can legitimise and accept social action (van Dijk, 1988) and it is through discourse that ideologies are reproduced, reinforced, and, in particular situations, replaced.

4. Finally, we assume that text—the product of what one says or writes—is intertextual. Texts are full of other texts, accessing them for stylistic, ironic effects, or ideological messages. Intertextuality can be intentional, but it also can be unwitting; this suggests that certain texts have a dominant role in how certain contents or experiences are constructed.

We firmly situate the methodological perspective of this book in the qualitative research paradigm. We take a bottom-up, 'insider' perspective. We want to look at the reality of suicide and its process through the eyes of those who were about to take their lives. Moreover, the core of our endeavour is firmly based on the analysis of the lexico-grammatical structures of language, which can be repeated and reproduced. In this way, qualitative research brings us closer to the perspective of the person we study, setting aside the issue of the researcher's perspective being imposed on the studied reality (Hammersley, 2008; Bloor, 2001).

Finally, Critical Discourse Analysis is interested in at least seven dimensions of discourse:

- properties of 'naturally occurring' language use (i.e., as used by real language users instead of abstract language systems and invented examples);
- larger units than isolated words and sentences and, hence, new basic units of analysis: texts, discourses, conversations, speech acts, or communicative events;
- the extension of linguistics beyond sentence grammar and towards a study of action and interaction;
- the extension to non-verbal (semiotic, multimodal, visual) aspects of interaction and communication: gestures, images, film, the internet, and multimedia;
- dynamic (socio)-cognitive or interactional moves and strategies;
- functions of (social, cultural, situative, and cognitive) contexts of language use;
- text grammar and language use: coherence, anaphora, topics, macrostructures, speech acts, interactions, turn-taking, signs, politeness, argumentation, rhetoric, mental models (Wodak & Meyer, 2016, p. 2).

### *Analysing Agency*

In this section, we briefly present what it means to analyse 'doing things' in discourse. Our analyses are informed particularly by the linguistics of Halliday (1994) who sees it in terms of the linguistically represented participant engaged in a process, that is, who was involved in what kind of action? We understand, of course, that the linguistic agent might not necessarily be the 'sociological' one (van Leeuwen, 2008), that is to say, as one who is taken to be an agent in a particular social context. However, assuming that the linguistic form is a socially underpinned way of structuring the world, it is the language and its form, used in a particular context, that are the foundation for any discussion of representation.

Halliday's systemic-functional grammar sees language as a meaning-making system with an emphasis on choice and proposes 'transitivity' as a grammar of experience (Halliday, 1985; 1978; Halliday & Hasan, 1985). Transitivity, part of the 'ideational metafunction', is a resource for constructing our experience of extralinguistic reality in terms of configurations of a process, participants, and circumstances (Martin, Matthiessen, & Painter, 1997), that is, in terms of who does what to whom, when, where, and how? Language enables its users to build a picture of reality and thereby make sense of their experience. Through transitivity, language affords its users grammatical structures through which they focus on the processes around them (Halliday, 1985).

Borrowing from Halliday's basic model of representing reality—which consists of a participant (normally rendered by nouns or pronouns), the process ascribed to the participant (normally rendered by a verb), and the circumstances in which it happens—we assume that the basic representation of the act of suicide is something like:

**participant–process–in circumstances.**

In other words, the basic representation of extralinguistic reality can be rendered by a sentence such as, 'A person does (something) somewhere/some time'. It is the first two elements, the participant and the process, that are indispensable in representation, although different languages render them differently. Halliday (1994) makes a distinction between six types of processes:

- Material processes refer to doing, happening, creating, and changing. Such processes are used to refer to stereotypical actions (e.g., kicking, walking, hitting).
- Mental processes refer to feeling, thinking, or seeing (e.g., considering, reminiscing, noticing).

- Relational processes refer to being and having an attribute or identity (e.g., being nice, being away).
- Behavioural processes refer to behaving (e.g. laughing, smiling, signing).
- Verbal processes are those referring to all those actions that are about saying something (e.g., promising, talking, warning).
- Existential processes relate to existing and being there, such as in the sentence, 'There are lions in Africa.'

As we write this chapter, our native Poland and other countries in Central Europe have been experiencing catastrophic flooding. Consider a hypothetical report in which one news report says something like, 'The flood water is tearing buildings down', while another, however, is telling us, 'I saw the flood water tear buildings down.' Yet another says: 'People say the flood water tore buildings down.' There are considerable differences between the three reports, and it has to do with the use of material, mental and verbal processes, and the agency they render. Only the first one renders reality in terms of agency and answers a hypothetical question such as, 'What happened there?' The others are answers to questions such as: 'What did you see?' and 'What do people say?' respectively.

It is worth pointing out that there might be more participants than only the one acting. When an actor is kicking, they are likely to be kicking something. And so, the other participant is the object of kicking or its goal. When the goal is human, we sometimes refer to the goal as the patient.

Consider two sentences such as:

1. I broke the vase (actor + process + goal).
2. The vase broke (actor + process).

There is a significant difference between the two sentences. In the first one, the actor is the agent, the doer. In the other sentence, the actor is an affected participant, someone or something that has things happen to them. Here, the analysis in terms of transitivity is helped by what is often called an ergative analysis, which is predominantly concerned with causality in actions.

### *Critical Discourse Analysis and Health Communication*

As Critical Discourse Analysis (CDA) is concerned with power relations and ideological foundations of discourse, it is capable of responding to calls for more attention to the role of language and power in healthcare, clinical encounters, and patients' experiences of health and illness that have been made over the last three decades or so (e.g., Mishler, 1984; Frank, 1995). And yet, contrary to other approaches to discourse (Georgaca, 2014; see also an earlier account by Harper, 1995), the topic of health, and in particular, mental health, has received relatively scant attention in the critical study of discourse.

Discourse analytic studies of mental health (for somatic health, see a review by Koteyko, 2014; also Wodak, 1997) are seldom frequent and focus on three main areas: (1) representations of mental disorders and those suffering from them; (2) experiences of the ill, their families, and personnel; and (3) medical/therapeutic communication.[1]

In the first of these themes, researchers focus on mainstream media (Bilić & Georgaca, 2007), social media (Clarke & Ameron, 2015), medical texts (e.g., Crowe, 2000) or policy documents (Callaghan, Fellin, & Warner-Gale, 2017). The two most commonly identified and analysed discourses in media are those of dangerousness and bio-medicalisation (e.g., Bilić & Georgaca, 2007). In addition, discourse analysts focus on representations of mental disorders in psychiatric discourses, both the ICD and DSM (e.g., Crowe, 2000; Freedman & Honkasilta, 2017).

The second thematic strand in Critical Discourse research focuses on the experiences of patients, their close ones, and medical personnel. For example, there is research on illness experience (Wilson & Crowe, 2009; Galasiński, 2008; 2013) and social identities (Ziółkowska & Galasiński, 2017; Jones et al., 2016). Finally, there is also research into medical documentation. Although medical documentation is the subject of some research, this is the least explored issue and CDA has barely engaged with it at all. While there is some research on medical notes in non-text-based discourse analysis (Berring, Pedersen, & Buss, 2015), we are aware of only one text-based study into medical notes in mental health settings (Galasiński & Ziółkowska, 2017).

### *Qualitative Suicidology*

Our final methodological point is about the relationship between discourse analysis and suicidology. We locate our research in the qualitative suicidological strand, which, although still on the margins, is rapidly growing. Despite that suicidologists stress the importance of methodological diversity, which would lead to a greater understanding of suicide and suicidal behaviour (e.g., Rogers & Apel, 2010; Leenaars, 2002), bottom-up approaches in suicide research are marginal (e.g., Hjelmeland, 2016).

Although qualitative suicidology has been developing rapidly, suicidology continues to be almost exclusively quantitative. Suicidological research can be grouped into three kinds of research: epidemiological, biological, and interventionist (Hjelmeland & Knizek, 2010). These kinds of research account for 97% of articles published in three leading journals in suicidology: *Archives of Suicide Research*, *Crisis*, and *Suicide and*

*Life-threatening Behavior* (Hjelmeland & Knizek, 2010; also Goldblatt et al., 2012; White et al., 2016). The only three book-length suicidological studies that report qualitative research are our recent books (Ziółkowska, 2016; Galasiński, 2017; Galasiński & Ziółkowska, 2020).

The dominant perspective in suicidology sees suicide as static and individual, probably resulting from mental illness and associated with identifiable risk factors, which became the main focal point of suicidological endeavours (White 2017; White et al., 2016). Inevitably, suicide is seen outside its social context, let alone its meaning, always to be prevented and controlled. This perspective was solidified in a recent declaration from the editor of a leading suicidological journal, who stated that only the quantitative perspective could lead to progress in suicidological research (Joiner, 2011).

And yet, there is a growing unease within mainstream suicidology. Rogers and Lester (2010) point out that after producing volumes of work, understanding suicide is still elusive. Fitzpatrick (2011) suggests that insight into narratively constructed experience is crucial for extending suicidological knowledge of meanings of suicide in its social context. Lester and Stack (2015; also Hjelmeland, 2016) reinforce this message by saying that the mere correlation of different variables does not bring suicidology closer to understanding suicide. They also call for more qualitative research.

In our view, the most interesting counterpoint to the mainstream suicidological view of suicide comes from the critical suicidological perspective. In contrast to mainstream suicidology, its critical counterpart suggests engagement with the social anchoring of suicide, and, in particular, seeing it within social, historical, cultural, and political contexts. Suicide no longer becomes an object for uncomplicated scientific inspection, but an event that is socially entangled (Kirmayer, 2012; Marsh, 2010; White & Kral, 2014; White 2017). White (2017) argues that critical suicidology introduces doubt into what the mainstream takes for granted. The self is no longer taken as the sole agent naturally doing away with its existence (see Jaworski, 2014), while at the same time, it poses questions as to the inevitable positioning of suicide as unjustified and to be stopped (Button, 2016; consider also the notion of rational suicide, Richards, 2017; Werth, 1999; Mayo, 1986).

The two approaches should not be seen as separate from each other, though. Indeed, a recent critique of the most prevalent theory of suicide (Hjelmeland & Knizek, 2020) resulted in a defence of the Interpersonal theory of suicide (Klonsky, 2019; Smith et al., 2019), and, more importantly, in an attempt to offer a platform for joining up the two approaches. Abrutyn and Mueller (2019) explicitly focus on the narrow understanding of science in mainstream suicidology and postulate the inclusion of the 'softer' qualitative perspective into the dominant research perspective.

In this book, we hope to reinforce the qualitative platform for a study of suicide and, in a way, offer a new insight into the experience and meaning of suicide (see Boldt, 1988; Colucci, 2013). If Lester (2000) was right that suicidology had reached its end and needed innovation (also Rogers & Lester, 2010; Rogers & Apel, 2010; Rogers, 2003), we hope this volume will strengthen the new perspective.

We see discourse analysis as capable of responding to calls for understanding the individuality of suicide in its social and cultural context (Munster & Broz, 2015). This is seconded by Marsh (2010; 2016) and Fullagar (2003) who argue that the current psychiatric and suicidological discourses distance researchers—by pathologising suicide—from suicide as an embodied social act (for a critique of scientism, see Fitzpatrick, 2015 and Hjelmeland & Knizek, 2011; for a social perspective, see Roen, Scourfield, & McDermott, 2008). Discourse analysis offers a much more holistic view and understanding of suicide through the perspective of those who constructed it in their suicide notes (see also Gavin & Rogers, 2006).

## The Data

There are three sets of data this book is based on, two sets of interviews and a set of suicide notes. The first is a set of 65 semi-structured interviews conducted in 16 wards in four hospitals in the south and southwest of Poland. They were conducted with patients who had been admitted to hospital after a suicide attempt. Of the interviewees 36 were male and 29 were female. The interviews lasted from 7 to 115 minutes and the mean duration was 28 minutes.[2]

The data collection was performed in accordance with the Declaration of Helsinki, with ethical approvals obtained from the ethics committee of the University of Social Sciences and Humanities in Poland. The participants received written information regarding the scope of the research, the identity and contact details of the researchers, the opportunity to withdraw from the studies at any point with no consequence, their confidentiality and anonymity, and all other information as required under Polish policies for research in a clinical context.

The second interview set was collected between October 2018 and December 2018. We interviewed 22 participants, 11 participants being male, and 11 being female. They were patients hospitalised after a suicide attempt. The data were collected in psychiatric hospital during their first days in the hospital. The interviews lasted between 8 and 86 minutes and the mean duration was 35 minutes. Similar to the first corpus of the data, the study was performed in accordance with the Declaration of Helsinki, with ethical approvals obtained from the Ethics Committee of the University of Social Sciences and Humanities in Poland. The participants received written information regarding the scope of the research, identity and contact details of the researchers, the opportunity to withdraw from the studies at any point with no consequence, their confidentiality and anonymity, and all other information as required in accordance with Polish policies for research in clinical contexts.

We have chosen not to represent our informants with fictional initials, let alone fictional first names as often is the practice in the literature. This is for two reasons. The stories we cite carry with them some sensitive details—we did not wish to create the possibility of false identities. Second, the default address form for adults in Polish is the polite form *pan/pani* (the equivalent of German *Sie* or Spanish *usted*) and referring to informants, adult people, only by first names (fictional or not) could be seen as patronising and to a certain extent, at least, puts them in a position of lower or inferior status, something our informants, and probably most other people with mental illness, have to struggle with daily.

Moreover, throughout the book, we generally refer to the individuals we interviewed as 'informants' or 'participants', rather than as 'patients'. This is because the narratives they offered concerned non-clinical issues. When the context warrants it, we refer to them as patients (rather than, clients, service users, or survivors; see: Costa et al., 2019). We realise that this is not an 'innocent' choice; there is a substantial body of literature on the stigmatisation of mental health users (for reviews, see, Hayward & Bright, 1997; Rüsch, Angermeyer, & Corrigan, 2005), their social and political isolation (Erdner et al., 2005; Kelly, 2006) and particularly the role of labelling in stigmatisation (Corrigan, Kerr, & Knudsen, 2005). Indeed, several studies were carried out into the very use of the expression 'mental patient', finding negative associations invoked by it (Johannsen, 1969; Rabkin, 1972). Also, we are mindful of Speed's (2006) analysis of self-labelling on the spectrum of patients–customers–survivors, pointing out that it might reflect the position between passive acceptance and active resistance to the mental health system.

Still, we have made our choice precisely because our informants used the word 'patient' to refer to themselves. Also, we think that Speed's (2006) argument is somewhat tendentious in that he does not consider the possibility that accepting one's patienthood might be part of accepting one's illness (Davidson, 2003; Morse & Johnson, 1991) and part of a route towards recovery. It might also be part of 'coming out' and challenging the stigma (Corrigan & Matthews, 2003). We make these choices, also, as we reject the argument that uniform resistance towards psychiatric services is universally good or desirable. It can be counterproductive.

All interviews were digitally recorded and later transcribed; the basis of our analyses are transcriptions. In qualitative research, the transcription of spoken data is considered significant, going beyond simple data processing (Atkinson & Heritage, 1984). We adopted a simplified version of the Jeffersonian system (i.e., Jefferson, 2004). The system allowed us to accurately render the contents and form of the informants' responses, while controlling the level of information needed for our analysis and ensuring transparency (Hepburn & Bolden, 2017).

The third set of data is the Polish Corpus of Suicide Notes (*Polski korpus listów pożegnalnych samobójców*; www.pcsn.uni.wroc.pl/). It contains authentic suicide notes collected from regional prosecutors' offices in Poland in 2008. Only notes from people who committed suicided were put in the corpus (for a detailed account and description of the corpus, its subcorpora, and the process of data collection, see Zaśko-Zielińska, 2013).

The corpus contains 614 suicide notes, written between 1998 and 2008. Of those notes, 456 (74%) were written by 290 men, while the remaining 256 notes were written by 92 women. The youngest author of a suicide note in the corpus was 12 (a girl), and the oldest was 89 (a man). The corpus contains information about the time and the place of writing (finding), the age of the author, their gender and the medium (599 notes were handwritten), and sometimes about their marital status.

We only had access to the processed version of the notes. In other words, we worked on digitised and fully anonymised texts of the notes, with no access to their material original or their facsimiles. The only aspect of the notes preserved in the corpus was the use of capital letters. We have preserved the capitalisation in the Polish versions of the notes, which we have put in the appendices after every chapter. We have also preserved the spelling, punctuation, and layout of the text as it was presented in the corpus.

All the data we have are in Polish. Do we therefore write about Polish suicide notes or Polish interviews? There is no evidence of significant national differences at least in the contents of suicide notes (indeed, suicide notes seem to have considerable similarities regardless of who wrote them and where they wrote them), including those written in Poland. Indeed, Barbagli (2015) suggests that there is a 'Western' attitude towards suicide. Alternatively, we do not know of any cross-cultural studies of interviews with people after suicide attempts. Perhaps our book will give rise to such research in the future. We would speculate, however, that perhaps, since the notes are written at the most dramatic moment of a person's life, and the stories we collected are about this very dramatic moment, the differences between certain identities fade away.

Finally, in the discussions we refer to our translations of the Polish originals. We attempted to render not only the content of the Polish originals, but also its 'flavour' and 'gist'. Sometimes, it resulted in disjointed or 'bad' English; sometimes the language was barely intelligible. This is because the Polish originals were like that. Occasionally, we offered some information in square brackets (especially noting text that was removed to maintain the anonymity of the authors). Moreover, we also decided against using any contractions in the English translations. Contrary to English, Polish does not use contractions, and their imposition on the translations would, in our view, be too interpretative. We do realise, however, that just as the presence of contractions carries meaning, their absence does too, and some of the English translations may seem unduly formal and stilted. Unfortunately, this could not be avoided. In most cases, we introduced punctuation to the English translations. We also understand that it may offer an interpretation of the Polish originals, but it also makes them more intelligible. Importantly, all our analyses were carried out on the Polish originals.

## Vocabulary

Speaking of suicide is now underpinned by considerable discussions. The Centers for Disease Control and Prevention (CDC) announced a glossary of terms that should be used when referring to suicide and suicidal behaviour. Their effort is as much positive in recommending the use of certain terms (such as 'suicide' or 'suicide attempt') as it is negative in that they recommend not using several expressions. Thus, phrases such as 'completed suicide', 'failed attempt', and 'successful suicide' are all deemed unacceptable (see Crosby et al., 2011; Posner et al., 2007). We think that such proposals are uncontentious.

The other initiative is more controversial in our view, and it concerns the use of the phrase 'commit suicide'. We offer a fulsome discussion on the use of the phrase in Chapter 2. Here, we just would like to flag the issue. The point against the use of the phrase that is often made is that the verb 'commit' places suicide very firmly in the legal, criminalised domain. It suggests that suicide is a crime, and since suicide is not one, 'commit' should be avoided.

This is a significant oversimplification as the verb, admittedly not too often, can collocate with positive events, as in the phrase 'commit an act of bravery'. Indeed, such discussions concern only English and do not exist for example in Polish, where the phrase *popełnić samobojstwo* ('commit suicide') could be said to have similar connotations. More importantly, neither academics, nor activists should usurp the right to control the language people use, especially those who have experienced the tragedy of suicide of a close one or, indeed, their attempt.

Moreover, as we argue in Chapter 2, the key problem is that the new preferred phrase 'die by suicide' takes away the agency behind suicide. People do not just 'die by suicide', they do things to kill themselves. Phrases such as 'take one's life' or 'kill oneself', in turn, do not mention the word 'suicide'. To a considerable extent, we think the issue has no solution. In our book, we tend to speak of killing oneself and taking one's life, but we also use the phrase 'commit suicide', mostly because people we talked to also used it. To repeat, it is not for us to make value judgements on their choices.

## Overview of the Book

Our book consists of two parts. In the first part, we are interested in how people engaged in suicidal action position themselves in the act. We look at the stories of the self in suicide. The second part of the book looks at the stories of the self in relationships.

We start with a chapter on how the self and its agency are positioned in two discourses. First, we explore how suicide and its relationship with the self are constructed in institutional discourse. We argue that institutional discourses, both medical and activist, remove the person from their accounts of suicide. Suicide happens and is not done, or, indeed, committed. We juxtapose these results with people's stories. In contrast to institutional representations, the stories of lived experiences show different relevancies. In such narratives, the nature of suicide is hidden, while the individual's agency is preserved.

In Chapter 3, we examine constructions of agency in reference to the individual engaged in suicidal action. We are interested in the stories of what the person who is about to take their life does when engaging in suicide action. We extend our argument that understanding suicide only as a person's death is unhelpful as most definitions of suicide propose. But we also want to see how agency is constructed in reference to the time around the suicidal act. Thus, building on our earlier work on the suicidal process and the agency within it, we are interested in accounts of waiting for death as part of the process of taking one's own life. Interestingly, it is precisely at the margins that representations of agency are at their most unambiguous.

In Chapter 4, the last in the first section, we discuss ways in which suicide is romanticised in suicide notes. We are interested in all those stories in suicide letters in which suicide is represented as leading to positive, good, and beautiful outcomes. Such stories put the person taking their life at the very centre of such beauty about which the whole world should learn.

The second part of the book is where we explore narrated relationships in which the suicidal individual finds themself. In contrast to the dominant views of suicide in which suicide starts in the individual, we want to show that such views oversimplify matters. Relationships are often at the centre of a suicide story.

In Chapter 5, we show that those engaged in suicidal action consistently position themselves and their act in a relationship with their close ones. We argue that suicide is positioned as affecting people who are left behind. More significantly, we also show that suicide is represented as not affecting the existing relationships. Time and again, writers of suicide notes constructed their relationships as surviving their suicide. Alternatively, our informants in ex-post-facto interviews positioned their relationships as important for the future. The regrets they told us about were related to their close ones, who at the same time offered perspectives for the future.

Chapter 6 explores constructions of relationships in suicide notes written by parents and explicitly addressed to their children. We are primarily interested in how the writing parent represents their relationship with their child, but also how their relationships with the other parent and other significant people are constructed. Chapter 7 complements these discussions with an account of parents' legacy. On the one hand, we discussed the grand legacy suicide—positioned as a path towards a desirable outcome. In some cases, suicide is committed for the outcomes to be brought about. On the other hand, we discussed the little legacies. These were messages of advice—the last words of wisdom from the dying parent. We also discussed the last messages of care, for example, the dying parents expressing continuing love and presence.

In the last of the empirical chapters, Chapter 8, we are concerned with constructions of love in suicide notes. We are interested in how love is represented in the last farewells. However, we also want to analyse love in the narratives following a suicide attempt. We argue that suicide letters are aimed at creating a bond between the writer and addressee, a bond that in some cases is intended to last beyond the suicide with a love that should be reciprocated.

## Notes

1 Our account is a precis of our earlier review (Galasiński & Ziółkowska, 2021).
2 The data were collected between July 2013 and October 2015 within two projects supported by the National Science Centre in Poland (SONATA 2012/05/D/HS6/02390 and OPUS 2013/09/B/HS6/02796).

## References

Abrutyn, S., & Mueller, A. S. (2019). Toward a robust science of suicide: Epistemological, theoretical, and methodological considerations in advancing suicidology. *Death Studies, 45*(7), 522–527. https://doi.org/10.1080/07481187.2019.1660081

American Foundation for Suicide Prevention [AFSP]. (2024). *Suicide statistics.* Retrieved from: https://afsp.org/about-suicide/suicide-statistics/

American Psychiatric Association [APA] (2013). *Diagnostic and Statistical Manual of Mental Disorders, Fifth Edition* (DSM-5). American Psychiatric Association Publishing.
American Psychiatric Association [APA]. (2022). *Diagnostic and Statistical Manual of Mental Disorders, Fifth Edition, Text Revision* (DSM-5-TR). American Psychiatric Association Publishing.
Atkinson, J. M., & Heritage, J. (1984). *Structures of social action: Studies in conversation analysis*. Cambridge University Press.
Baams, L., Grossman, A. H., & Russell, S. T. (2015). Minority stress and mechanisms of risk for depression and suicidal ideation among lesbian, gay, and bisexual youth. *Developmental Psychology, 51*(5), 688–696. https://doi.org/10.1037/a0038994
Bantjes, J., & Swartz, L. (2019). 'What can we learn from first-person narratives?' The case of nonfatal suicidal behavior. *Qualitative Health Research, 29*(10), 1497–1507. https://doi.org/10.1177/1049732319832869
Barbagli, M. (2015). *Farewell to the world: A history of suicide*. Polity Press.
Barker, C., & Galasiński, D. (2001). *Cultural studies and discourse analysis*. Sage.
Battin, M. P. (1995). *Ethical issues in suicide*. Prentice-Hall, Inc.
Baumeister, R. F. (1990). Suicide as escape from self. *Psychological Review, 97*(1), 90–113. https://doi.org/10.1037/0033-295X.97.1.90
Belsher, B. E., Smolenski, D. J., Pruitt, L. D., Bush, N. E., Beech, E. H., Workman, D. E., Morgan, R. L., Evatt, D. P., Tucker, J., & Skopp, N. A. (2019). Prediction models for suicide attempts and deaths: A systematic review and simulation. *JAMA Psychiatry, 76*(6), 642–651. https://doi.org/10.1001/jamapsychiatry.2019.0174
Benson, O., Gibson, S., Boden, Z. V., & Owen, G. (2016). Exhausted without trust and inherent worth: A model of the suicide process based on experiential accounts. *Social Science & Medicine, 163*, 126–134. https://doi.org/10.1016/j.socscimed.2016.06.045
Berring, L. L., Pedersen, L., & Buus, N. (2015). Discourses of aggression in forensic mental health: A critical discourse analysis of mental health nursing staff records. *Nursing Inquiry, 22*(4), 296–305. https://doi.org/10.1111/nin.12113
Bertolote, J. M., Fleischmann, A., De Leo, D., & Wasserman, D. (2003). Suicide and mental disorders: Do we know enough? *The British Journal of Psychiatry, 183*(5), 382–383. https://doi.org/10.1192/bjp.183.5.382
Bilić, B., & Georgaca, E. (2007). Representations of 'mental illness' in Serbian newspapers: A critical discourse analysis. *Qualitative Research in Psychology, 4*(1–2), 167–186. https://doi.org/10.1080/14780880701473573
Billig, M., Condor, S., Edwards, D., Gane, M., Middleton, D., & Radley, A. R. (1988). *Ideological dilemmas*. Sage.
Bloor, M. (2001). The ethnography of health and medicine. In P. Atkinson, A. Coffey, S. Delamont, J. Lofland, & L. Lofland (Eds.), *Handbook of ethnography* (pp. 177–187). Sage.
Boldt, M. (1988). The meaning of suicide: Implications for research. *Crisis: The Journal of Crisis Intervention and Suicide Prevention, 9*(2), 93–108.

Button, M. (2016). Suicide and social justice: Toward a political approach to suicide. *Political Research Quarterly*, *69*(2), 270–280. http://www.jstor.org/stable/44018009

Cairns, J. M., Graham, E., & Bambra, C. (2017). Area-level socioeconomic disadvantage and suicidal behaviour in Europe: A systematic review. *Social Science & Medicine*, *192*, 102–111. https://doi.org/10.1016/j.socscimed.2017.09.034

Callaghan, J. E., Fellin, L. C., & Warner-Gale, F. (2017). A critical analysis of Child and Adolescent Mental Health Services policy in England. *Clinical Child Psychology and Psychiatry*, *22*(1), 109–127. https://doi.org/10.1177/1359104516640318

Canetto, S. S. (2017). Suicide: Why are older men so vulnerable? *Men and Masculinities*, *20*(1), 49–70. https://doi.org/10.1177/1097184X15613832

Canetto, S. S., & Sakinofsky, I. (1998). The gender paradox in suicide. *Suicide and Life-Threatening Behavior*, *28*(1), 1–23. https://doi.org/10.1111/j.1943-278X.1998.tb00622.x

Chouliaraki, L., & Fairclough, N. (1999). *Discourse in late modernity*. Edinburgh University Press.

Clarke, J. N., & Van Ameron, G. (2015). Parents whose children have oppositional defiant disorder talk to one another on the internet. *Child and Adolescent Social Work Journal*, *32*(4), 341–350. https://doi.org/10.1007/s10560-015-0377-5

Colucci, E. (2013). Culture, cultural meaning(s), and suicide. In E. Colucci & D. Lester (Eds.), *Suicide and culture: Understanding the context* (pp. 25–46). Hogrefe Publishing.

Corrigan, P. W., Kerr, A., & Knudsen, L. (2005). The stigma of mental illness. *Applied and Preventive Psychology*, *11*(3), 179–190. https://doi.org/10.1016/j.appsy.2005.07.001

Corrigan, P. W., & Matthews, A. K. (2003). Stigma and disclosure. *Journal of Mental Health*, *12*(3), 235–248. https://doi.org/10.1080/0963823031000118221

Costa, D. S., Mercieca-Bebber, R., Tesson, S., Seidler, Z., & Lopez, A. L. (2019). Patient, client, consumer, survivor or other alternatives? A scoping review of preferred terms for labelling individuals who access healthcare across settings. *BMJ Open*, *9*(3), e025166. https://doi.org/10.1136/bmjopen-2018-025166

Crosby, A. E., Cheltenham, M. P., & Sacks, J. J. (1999). Incidence of suicidal ideation and behavior in the United States, 1994. *Suicide and Life-Threatening Behavior*, *29*(2), 131–140. https://doi.org/10.1111/j.1943-278X.1999.tb01051.x

Crosby, A. E., Ortega, L., & Melanson, C. (2011). *Self-directed violence surveillance: Uniform definitions and recommended data elements*. Centers for Disease Control and Prevention.

Crowe, M. (2000). Constructing normality: A discourse analysis of the DSM-IV. *Journal of Psychiatric and Mental Health Nursing*, *7*(1), 69–77. https://doi.org/10.1046/j.1365-2850.2000.00261.x

Davidson, L. (2003). *Living outside mental illness*. New York University Press.

De Leo, D. (2011). DSM-V and the future of suicidology. *Crisis*, *32*(5), 233–239. https://doi.org/10.1027/0227-5910/a000128

De Leo, D., Burgis, S., Bertolote, J. M., Kerkhof, A. J., & Bille-Brahe, U. (2006). Definitions of suicidal behavior: Lessons learned from the WHO/EURO Multicentre Study. *Crisis*, *27*(1), 4–15. https://doi.org/10.1027/0227-5910.27.1.4

Durkheim, E. (1897/1966). *Suicide: A study in sociology*. Free Press.

Erdner, A., Magnusson, A., Nystro, M., & Lütze, K. (2005). Social and existential alienation experienced by people with long-term mental illness. *Scandinavian Journal of Caring Sciences*, *19*(4), 373–380. https://doi.org/10.1111/j.1471-6712.2005.00364.x

Eurostat. (2024). *Deaths by suicide in the EU down by 13% in a decade*. Retrieved from: https://ec.europa.eu/eurostat/web/products-eurostat-news/w/edn-20240909-1

Fairclough, N. (1989). *Language and power*. Longman.

Fairclough, N. (1992). *Discourse and social change*. Polity Press.

Fairclough, N. (1995). *Critical discourse analysis*. Longman.

Fairclough, N. (2003). *Analysing discourse*. Routledge.

Fairclough, N., & Wodak, R. (1997). Critical discourse analysis. In T. A. van Dijk (Ed.), *Discourse as social interaction* (pp. 258–284). Sage.

Fehling, K. B., & Selby, E. A. (2021). Suicide in DSM-5: Current evidence for the proposed suicide behavior disorder and other possible improvements. *Frontiers in Psychiatry*, *11*, 499980. https://doi.org/10.3389/fpsyt.2020.499980

Fitzpatrick, S. (2011). Looking beyond the qualitative and quantitative divide: Narrative, ethics and representation in suicidology. *Suicidology Online*, *2*, 29–37.

Fitzpatrick, S. J. (2015). Scientism as a social response to the problem of suicide. *Journal of Bioethical Inquiry*, *12*(4), 613–622. https://doi.org/10.1007/s11673-015-9662-4

Fitzpatrick, S. J. (2016). Ethical and political implications of the turn to stories in suicide prevention. *Philosophy, Psychiatry, & Psychology*, *23*(3), 265–276. https://dx.doi.org/10.1353/ppp.2016.0029

Fowler, R. (1985). Power. In T. A. Van Dijk (Ed.), *Handbook of discourse analysis*, vol. 4 (pp. 61–82). Academic Press.

Fowler, R. (1991). *Language in the news*. Routledge.

Fowler, R. (1996). On critical linguistics. In R. C. Caldas-Coulthard & M. Coulthard (Eds.), *Texts and practices* (pp. 3–14). Routledge.

Fowler, R., Hodge, B., Kress, G., & Trew, T. (Eds.) (1979). *Language and control*. Routledge.

Frank, A. W. (1995). *The wounded story-teller*. University of Chicago Press.

Franklin, J. C., Ribeiro, J. D., Fox, K. R., Bentley, K. H., Kleiman, E. M., Huang, X., Musacchio, K. M., Jaroszewski, A. C., Chang, B. P., & Nock, M. K. (2017). Risk factors for suicidal thoughts and behaviors: A meta-analysis of 50 years of research. *Psychological Bulletin*, *143*(2), 187–232. https://doi.org/10.1037/bul0000084

Freedman, J. E., & Honkasilta, J. M. (2017). Dictating the boundaries of ab/normality: Acritical discourse analysis of the diagnostic criteria for attention deficit hyperactivity disorder and hyperkinetic disorder. *Disability & Society*, *32*(4), 565–588. https://doi.org/10.1080/09687599.2017.1296819

Fullagar, S. (2003). Wasted lives. The social dynamics of shame and youth suicide. *Journal of Sociology*, *39*(3), 291–307. https://doi.org/10.1177/0004869003035076
Galasiński, D. (2004). *Men and the language of emotions*. Palgrave.
Galasiński, D. (2008). *Men's discourses of depression*. Palgrave Macmillan.
Galasinski, D. (2013). *Fathers, fatherhood and mental illness: A discourse analysis of rejection*. Palgrave Macmillan.
Galasinski, D. (2017). *Discourses of men's suicide notes: A qualitative analysis*. Bloomsbury Publishing.
Galasiński, D., & Ziółkowska, J. (2017). Construction of suicidal ideation in medical records. *Death Studies*, *41*(8), 493–501. https://doi.org/10.1080/07481187.2017.1332910
Galasinski, D., & Ziółkowska, J. (2020). *Discursive constructions of the suicidal process*. Bloomsbury Publishing.
Galasiński, D., & Ziółkowska, J. (2021). Critical discourse studies: Mad, bad or nuisance? Discursive constructions of detained patients in Polish nursing notes. In G. Brooks & D. Hunt (Eds.), *Analysing health communication: Discourse approaches* (pp. 215–239). Springer International Publishing.
Gavin, M., & Rogers, A. (2006). Narratives of suicide in psychological autopsy: Bringing lay knowledge back in. *Journal of Mental Health*, *15*(2), 135–144. https://doi.org/10.1080/09638230600608735
Georgaca, E. (2014). Discourse analytic research on mental distress: A critical overview. *Journal of Mental Health*, 23(2), 55–61. https://doi.org/10.3109/09638237.2012.734648
Gergen, J. K. (1973). Social psychology as history. *Journal of Personality and Social Psychology*, *26*, 309–320. https://doi.org/10.1037/h0034436
Goldblatt, M. J., Schechter, M., Maltsberger, J. T., & Ronningstam, E. (2012). Comparison of journals of suicidology. *Crisis*, 33(5), 301–305. https://doi.org/10.1027/0227-5910/a000146
Goodfellow, B., Kõlves, K., & De Leo, D. (2019). Contemporary classifications of suicidal behaviors. *Crisis*, *41*(3), 179–186. https://doi.org/10.1027/0227-5910/a000622
Hacking, I. (1990). *The taming of chance*. Cambridge University Press.
Hall, S. (1981). Encoding/Decoding. In S. Hall, D. Hobson, A. Lowe, & P. Willis (Eds.), *Culture, media, language* (pp. 128–138). Hutchinson.
Hall, S. (1996). For Allon White: Metaphors of transformation. In D. Morley & D. K. Chen (Eds.), *Stuart Hall* (pp. 287–307). Routledge.
Hall, S. (1997). The work of representation. In S. Hall (Ed.), *Representation: Cultural representation and signifying practices* (pp. 13–74). Sage.
Halliday, M. A. K. (1978). *Language as social semiotic*. Edward Arnold.
Halliday, M. A. K. (1994). *An introduction to functional grammar* (2nd ed.). Edward Arnold.
Halliday, M. A. K., & Hasan, R. (1985). *Language, context, and text*. Oxford University Press.
Hammersley, M. (2008). *Questioning qualitative inquiry: Critical essays*. Sage
Harper, D. (1995). Discourse analysis and 'mental health'. *Journal of Mental Health*, *4*, 347–357

Harré, R. (1979). *Social being: A theory for social psychology*. Blackwell.
Harris, E. C., & Barraclough, B. (1997). Suicide as an outcome for mental disorders. A meta-analysis. *The British Journal of Psychiatry*, *170*(3), 205–228. https://doi.org/10.1192/bjp.170.3.205
Hayward, P., & Bright, J. A. (1997). Stigma and mental illness. *Journal of Mental Health*, 6(4), 345–54. https://doi.org/10.1080/09638239718671
Hecht, J. M. (2013). *Stay. A history of suicide and the arguments against it*. Yale University Press.
Hengartner, M. P., Amendola, S., Kaminski, J. A., Kindler, S., Bschor, T., & Plöderl, M. (2021). Suicide risk with selective serotonin reuptake inhibitors and other new-generation antidepressants in adults: A systematic review and meta-analysis of observational studies. *Journal of Epidemiology and Community Health*, *75*, 523–530. https://doi.org/10.1136/jech-2020-214611
Henry, A. F., & Short, J. F. (1964). *Suicide and homicide: Some economic, sociological and psychological aspects of aggression*. Free Press.
Hepburn, A., & Bolden, G. (2013). The conversation analytic approach to transcription. In T. Stivers & J. Sidnell (Eds.). *The Blackwell handbook of conversation analysis* (pp. 57–76). Blackwell.
Hjelmeland, H. (2016). A critical look at current suicide research. In J. White, I. Marsh, M. Kral, & J. Morris (Eds.), *Critical suicidology. Transforming suicide research and prevention for the 21st century* (pp. 31–55). UBC Press.
Hjelmeland, H., & Knizek, B. L. (2010). Why we need qualitative research in suicidology. *Suicide and Life-Threatening Behavior*, *40*(1), 74–80. https://doi.org/10.1521/suli.2010.40.1.74
Hjelmeland, H., & Knizek, B. L. (2011). Methodology in suicidological research-contribution to the debate. *Suicidology Online*, *2*, 8–10.
Hjelmeland, H., & Knizek, B. L. (2020). The emperor's new clothes? A critical look at the interpersonal theory of suicide. *Death Studies*, *44*(3), 168–178. https://doi.org/10.1080/07481187.2018.1527796
Hodge, R., & Kress, G. (1988). *Social semiotics*. Polity Press.
Hodge, R., & Kress, G. (1993). *Language as ideology*. Routledge.
Hołówka, J. (2001). *Etyka w działaniu [Ethics in action]*. Prószyński i S-ka.
Huang, X., Harris, L. M., Funsch, K. M., Fox, K. R., & Ribeiro, J. D. (2022). Efficacy of psychotropic medications on suicide and self-injury: A meta-analysis of randomized controlled trials. *Translational Psychiatry*, *12*(1), 400. https://doi.org/10.1038/s41398-022-02173-9
Hudzik, T. J., & Cannon, K. E. (2014). Introduction. In K. E. Cannon & T. J. Hudzik (Eds.), *Suicide: Phenomenology and neurobiology* (pp. 1–7). Springer.
Imberton, G. (2012). Chol understandings of suicide and human agency. *Culture, Medicine, and Psychiatry*, *36*, 245–263. https://doi.org/10.1007/s11013-012-9252-4
Jaworski, K. (2014). *The gender of suicide: Knowledge production, theory and suicidology*. Ashgate Publishing Limited.
Jefferson, G. (2004). Glossary of transcript symbols with an introduction. In G. H. Lerner (Ed.), *Conversation analysis: Studies from the first generation* (pp. 13–31). John Benjamins.

Johannsen, W. J. (1969). Attitudes towards mental patients. *Mental Hygiene, 25*, 218–228.
Johnson, B. D. (1965). Durkheim's one cause of suicide. *American Sociological Review, 30*(6), 875–886. https://doi.org/10.2307/2090966
Joiner, T. E. (2005). *Why people die by suicide.* Harvard University Press.
Joiner, T. E., Jr. (2011). Editorial: Scientific rigor as the guiding heuristic for SLTB's editorial stance. *Suicide and Life-Threatening Behavior, 41*(5), 471–73. https://doi.org/10.1111/j.1943-278X.2011.00056.x
Jones, M., Pietilä, I., Joronen, K., Simpson, W., Gray, S., & Kaunonen, M. (2016). Parents with mental illness – a qualitative study of identities and experiences with support services. *Journal of Psychiatric and Mental Health Nursing, 23*(8), 471–478. https://doi.org/10.1111/jpm.12321
Kelly, B. D. (2006). The power gap: Freedom, power and mental illness. *Social Science & Medicine, 63*, 2118–2128. https://doi.org/10.1016/j.socscimed.2006.05.015
Kirmayer, L. J. (2012). Cultural competence and evidence-based practice in mental health: Epistemic communities and the politics of pluralism. *Social Science & Medicine, 75*(2), 249–256. https://doi.org/10.1016/j.socscimed.2012.03.018
Klonsky, E. D. (2019). The role of theory for understanding and preventing suicide (but not predicting it): A commentary on Hjelmeland and Knizek. *Death Studies, 44*(7), 459–462. https://doi.org/10.1080/07481187.2019.1594005
Klonsky, E. D., May, A. M., & Saffer, B. Y. (2016). Suicide, suicide attempts, and suicidal ideation. *Annual Review of Clinical Psychology, 12*(1), 307–330. https://doi.org/10.1146/annurev-clinpsy-021815-093204
Koteyko, N. (2014). Critical studies of health and illness discourses. In C. Hart & P. Cap (Eds.), *Contemporary critical discourse studies* (pp. 543–557). Bloomsbury.
Kress, G. R., & Van Leeuwen, T. (1996). *Reading images: The grammar of visual design.* Routledge.
Krzyżanowski, M., & Frochtner, B. (2016) Theories and concepts in critical discourse studies. *Discourse and Society, 27*, 253–61. https://doi.org/10.1177/0957926516630900
Kutchins, H., & Kirk, S. A. (1999). *Making us crazy.* Constable.
Leenaars, A. A. (2002). In defense of the idiographic approach: Studies of suicide notes and personal documents. *Archives of Suicide Research, 6*(1), 19–30. https://doi.org/10.1080/13811110213125
Lester, D. (2000). *Why people kill themselves: A 2000 summary of research on suicide (4th ed.).* Charles C Thomas Publisher.
Lester, D., & Stack, S. (Eds.). (2015). *Suicide as a dramatic performance.* Transaction Publishers.
MacDonald, M. (1989). The medicalization of suicide in England: Laymen, physicians, and cultural change, 1500–1870. *The Milbank Quarterly, 67*(1), 69–91. https://doi.org/10.2307/3350186
Mäki, N., & Martikainen, P. (2012). A register-based study on excess suicide mortality among unemployed men and women during different levels of unemployment in Finland. *J Epidemiol Community Health, 66*(4), 302–307. https://doi.org/10.1136/jech.2009.105908

Maris, R. W. (2015). *Pillaged. Psychiatric medications and suicide risk*. The University of South Carolina Press.

Marsh, I. (2010). *Suicide: Foucault, history and truth*. Cambridge University Press.

Marsh, I. (2013). The uses of history in the unmaking of modern suicide. *Journal of Social History, 46*(3), 744–756.

Marsh, I. (2016). Critiquing contemporary suicidology. In J. White, I. Marsh, M. Kral, & J. Morris (Eds.), *Critical suicidology. Transforming suicide research and prevention for the 21st century* (pp. 15–30). UBC Press.

Martin, J. R., Matthiessen, C. M. I. M., & Painter, C. (1997). *Working with functional grammar*. Edward Arnold.

Mayo, D. J. (1986). The concept of rational suicide. *Journal of Medicine and Philosophy, 11*(2), 143–155. https://doi.org/10.1093/jmp/11.2.143

Meehan, P. J., Lamb, J. A., Saltzman, L. E., & O'Carroll, P. W. (1992). Attempted suicide among young adults: Progress toward a meaningful estimate of prevalence. *American Journal of Psychiatry, 149*(1), 41–44. https://doi.org/10.1176/ajp.149.1.41

Menz, F. (1989). Manipulation strategies in newspapers. In R. Wodak (Ed.), *Language, power and ideology* (pp. 227–249). John Benjamins.

Milner, A., Sveticic, J., & De Leo, D. (2013). Suicide in the absence of mental disorder? A review of psychological autopsy studies across countries. *International Journal of Social Psychiatry, 59*(6), 545–554. https://doi.org/10.1177/0020764012444259

Minois, G. (2001). *History of suicide: Voluntary death in western culture*. Johns Hopkins University Press.

Mishler, E. (1984). *The discourse of medicine: Dialectics of medical interviews*. Ablex.

Morse, J., & Johnson, J. J. (1991). Towards a theory of illness. In J. M. Morse & J. L. Johnson (Eds.), *The illness experience: Dimensions of suffering* (pp. 315–342). Sage.

Mościcki, E. K. (1997). Identification of suicide risk factors using epidemiologic studies. *Psychiatric Clinics of North America, 20*(3), 499–517. https://doi.org/10.1016/s0193-953x(05)70327-0

Munster, D. & Broz, L. (2015). The anthropology of suicide: Ethnography and the tension of agency. In L. Broz & D. Munster Eds.), *Suicide and agency: Anthropological perspectives on self- destruction, personhood, and power* (pp. 3–26). Abingdon: Routledge.

Münster, D., & Broz, L. (2016). The anthropology of suicide: Ethnography and the tension of agency. In L. Broz & D. Münster (Eds.), *Suicide and agency* (pp. 3–24). Routledge.

O'Carroll, P. W., Berman, A. L., Maris, R. W., Moscicki, E. K., Tanney, B. L., & Silverman, M. M. (1996). Beyond the tower of Babel: A nomenclature for suicidology. *Suicide and Life-Threatening Behavior, 26*(3), 237–252. https://doi.org/10.1111/j.1943-278X.1996.tb00609.x

O'Connor, R., & Sheehy, N. (2000). *Understanding suicidal behaviour*. BPS Books.

O'Connor R. C. (2011). The integrated motivational–volitional model of suicidal behavior. *Crisis, 32*(6), 295–298. https://doi.org/10.1027/0227-5910/a000120

Obegi, J. H. (2021). Is suicidality a mental disorder? Applying DSM-5 guidelines for new diagnoses. *Death Studies*, *45*(8), 638–650. https://doi.org/10.1080/07481187.2019.1671546

Oliffe, J. L., Broom, A., Kelly, M. T., Bottorff, J. L., Creighton, G. M., & Ferlatte, O. (2018). Men on losing a male to suicide: A gender analysis. *Qualitative Health Research*, *28*(9), 1383–1394. https://doi.org/10.1177/1049732318769600

Oliogu, E., & Ruocco, A. C. (2024). DSM-5 suicidal behavior disorder: A systematic review of research on clinical utility, diagnostic boundaries, measures, pathophysiology and interventions. *Frontiers in Psychiatry*, *15*, 1278230. https://doi.org/10.3389/fpsyt.2024.1278230

Phillips, M. R. (2010). Rethinking the role of mental illness in suicide. *American Journal of Psychiatry*, *167*(7), 731–733. https://doi.org/10.1176/appi.ajp.2010.10040589

Pitman, A., Krysinska, K., Osborn, D., & King, M. (2012). Suicide in young men. *The Lancet*, *379*(9834), 2383–2392. https://doi.org/10.1016/S0140-6736(12)60731-4

Pokorny, A. D. (1983). Prediction of suicide in psychiatric patients: Report of a prospective study. *Archives of General Psychiatry*, *40*(3), 249–257. https://doi.org/10.1001/archpsyc.1983.01790030019002

Pokorny, A. D. (1993). Suicide prediction revisited. *Suicide and Life-Threatening Behavior*, *23*(1), 1–10. https://doi.org/10.1111/j.1943-278X.1993.tb00273.x

Posner, K., Oquendo, M. A., Gould, M., Stanley, B., & Davies, M. (2007). Columbia Classification Algorithm of Suicide Assessment (C-CASA): Classification of suicidal events in the FDA's pediatric suicidal risk analysis of antidepressants. *The American Journal of Psychiatry*, *164*(7), 1035–1043. https://doi.org/10.1176/ajp.2007.164.7.1035

Pridmore, S. (2011). Medicalisation of suicide. *The Malaysian Journal of Medical Sciences*, *18*(4), 78–83.

Rabkin, J. G. (1972). Opinions about mental illness. *Psychological Bulletin*, *77*(3), 153–177. https://doi.org/10.1037/h0032341

Richards, N. (2017). Old age rational suicide. *Sociology Compass*, *11*(3), e12456. https://doi.org/10.1111/soc4.12456

Riera-Serra, P., Navarra-Ventura, G., Castro, A., Gili, M., Salazar-Cedillo, A., Ricci-Cabello, I., Roldán-Espínola, L., Coronado-Simsic, V., García-Toro, M., Gómez-Juanes, R., & Roca, M. (2024). Clinical predictors of suicidal ideation, suicide attempts and suicide death in depressive disorder: A systematic review and meta-analysis. *European Archives of Psychiatry and Clinical Neuroscience*, *274*(7), 1543–1563. https://doi.org/10.1007/s00406-023-01716-5

River, J., & Flood, M. (2021). Masculinities, emotions and men's suicide. *Sociology of Health & Illness*, *43*(4), 910–927. https://doi.org/10.1111/1467-9566.13257

Robison, M., Udupa, N. S., Rice, T. B., Wilson-Lemoine, E., Joiner, T. E., & Rogers, M. L. (2024). The interpersonal theory of suicide: State of the science. *Behavior Therapy*, *55*(6), 1158–1171. https://doi.org/10.1016/j.beth.2024.04.008

Roen, K., Scourfield, J., & McDermott, E. (2008). Making sense of suicide: A discourse analysis of young people's talk about suicidal subjecthood. *Social Science & Medicine*, *67*(12), 2089–2097. https://doi.org/10.1016/j.socscimed.2008.09.019

Rogers, J. R. (2003). The anatomy of suicidology: A psychological science perspective on the status of suicide research. *Suicide and Life-Threatening Behavior*, *31*(1), 9–20. https://doi.org/10.1521/suli.33.1.9.22783

Rogers, J. R., & Apel, S. (2010). Revitalizing suicidology: A call for mixed methods designs. *Suicidology Online*, *1*, 92–94.

Rogers, J. R., & Lester, D. (2010). *Understanding suicide: Why we don't and how we might*. Hogrefe.

Rüsch, N, Angermeyer, M. C., & Corrigan, P. W. (2005). Mental illness stigma. *European Psychiatry*, *20*(8), 529–539. https://doi.org/10.1016/j.eurpsy.2005.04.004

Schmutte, T., Costa, M., Hammer, P., & Davidson, L. (2021). Comparisons between suicide in persons with serious mental illness, other mental disorders, or no known mental illness: Results from 37 US states, 2003–2017. *Schizophrenia Research*, *228*, 74–82. https://doi.org/10.1016/j.schres.2020.11.058

Shahram, S. Z., Smith, M. L., Ben-David, S., Feddersen, M., Kemp, T. E., & Plamondon, K. (2021). Promoting 'zest for life': A systematic literature review of resiliency factors to prevent youth suicide. *Journal of Research on Adolescence*, *31*(1), 4–24. https://doi.org/10.1111/jora.12588

Sheehy, K., Noureen, A., Khaliq, A., Dhingra, K., Husain, N., Pontin, E. E., Cawley, R., & Taylor, P. J. (2019). An examination of the relationship between shame, guilt and self-harm: A systematic review and meta-analysis. *Clinical Psychology Review*, *73*, 101779. https://doi.org/10.1016/j.cpr.2019.101779

Shneidman, E. (1996). *The suicidal mind*. Oxford University Press.

Silverman, M. M., & De Leo, D. (2016). Why there is a need for an international nomenclature and classification system for suicide. *Crisis*, *37*(2), 83–87. https://doi.org/10.1027/0227-5910/a000419

Sinyor, M., Silverman, M., Pirkis, J., & Hawton, K. (2024). The effect of economic downturn, financial hardship, unemployment, and relevant government responses on suicide. *The Lancet Public Health*, *9*(10), e802–e806. https://doi.org/10.1016/S2468-2667(24)00152-X

Smith, M. M., Sherry, S. B., Chen, S., Saklofske, D. H., Mushquash, C., Flett, G. L., & Hewitt, P. L. (2018). The perniciousness of perfectionism: A meta-analytic review of the perfectionism–suicide relationship. *Journal of Personality*, *86*(3), 522–542. https://doi.org/10.1111/jopy.12333

Smith, P. N., Schuler, K., Fadoir, N., Marie, L., & Basu, N. (2019). Socio-ecological context and the interpersonal theory of suicide: A response to Hjelmeland & Knizek. *Death Studies*, *44*(9), 547–551. https://doi.org/10.1080/07481187.2019.1586799

Speed, E. (2006). Patients, consumers and survivors. *Social Science & Medicine*, *62*(1), 28–38. https://doi.org/10.1016/j.socscimed.2005.05.025

Titscher, S., Meyer, M., Wodak, R., & Vetter, E. (2000). *Methods of text and discourse analysis*. Sage.

Tondo, L. (2014). Brief history of suicide Western cultures. In S. H. Koslow, P. Ruiz, & C. B. Nemeroff (Eds.), *A concise guide to understanding suicide. Epidemiology, pathophysiology and prevention* (s. 3–12). Cambridge University Press.

Van Dijk, T. A. (1988). *News analysis.* Case Studies of International and National News in the Press. Lawrence.

Van Dijk, T. A. (1993). Principles of critical discourse analysis. *Discourse & Society, 4*, 249–283. https://doi.org/10.1177/0957926593004002006

Van Dijk, T. A. (1998). *Ideology.* Sage.

Van Leeuwen, T. (2008). *Discourse and practice. New tools for critical discourse analysis.* Oxford University Press.

Van Leeuwen, T., & Wodak, R. (1999). Legitimizing immigration control. *Discourse Studies, 1*, 83–118. https://doi.org/10.1177/1461445699001001005

Van Orden, K. A., Witte, T. K., Cukrowicz, K. C., Braithwaite, S. R., Selby, E. A., & Joiner Jr., T. E. (2010). The interpersonal theory of suicide. *Psychological Review, 117*(2), 575–600. https://doi.org/10.1037/a0018697

Wagner, B. M., Wong, S. A., & Jobes, D. A. (2002). Mental health professionals' determinations of adolescent suicide attempts. *Suicide and Life-Threatening Behavior, 32*(3), 284–300. https://doi.org/10.1521/suli.32.3.284.22178 (https://psycnet.apa.org/doi/10.1521/suli.32.3.284.22178)

Werth, J. L. (Ed.). (1999). *Contemporary perspectives on rational suicide.* Psychology Press.

White, J. (2017). What can critical suicidology do? *Death Studies, 41*(8), 472–480. https://doi.org/10.1080/07481187.2017.1332901

White, J., & Kral, M. (2014). Re-thinking youth suicide: Language, culture and power. *Journal of Social Action for Counseling and Psychology*, 6(1), 122–142. https://doi.org/10.33043/JSACP.6.1.122-142

White, J., Marsh, I., Kral, M. J., & Morris, J. (2016). Introduction: Rethinking suicide. In J. White, I. Marsh, M. Kral, & J. Morris (Eds.), *Critical suicidology. Transforming suicide research and prevention for the 21st century* (pp. 1–14). UBC Press.

World Health Organization [WHO]. (2019). *Suicide in the world.* Retrieved from: https://iris.who.int/bitstream/handle/10665/345946/9789240036703-eng.pdf?sequence=1

World Health Organization [WHO]. (2024). *Suicide.* Retrieved from: www.who.int/news-room/fact-sheets/detail/suicide

Williams, J. M. G. (2014). *Cry of pain. Understanding suicide and the suicidal mind* (3rd ed.). Piatkus.

Williams, J. M. G. (1997). *Cry of pain: Understanding suicide and self-harm.* Penguin.

Wilson, L., & Crowe, M. (2009). Parenting with a diagnosis bipolar disorder. *Journal of Advanced Nursing, 65*(4), 877–884. https://doi.org/10.1111/j.1365-2648.2008.04954.x

Wodak, R. (1997). Critical discourse analysis and the study of doctor–patient interaction. In B. L. Gunnarsson, P. Linell, & B. Nordberg (Eds.), *The construction of professional discourse* (pp. 173–200). Routledge.

Wodak, R. (1999). Critical discourse analysis at the end of the 20th century. *Research on Language and Social Interaction*, 32, 185–193. https://doi.org/10.1080/08351813.1999.9683622

Wodak, R., & Meyer, M. (Eds.). (2016). *Methods of critical discourse studies*. Sage.

Zaśko-Zielińska, M. (2013). *Listy pożegnalne: w poszukiwaniu lingwistycznych wyznaczników autentyczności tekstu* [Farewell letters: in search of linguistic indicators of text authenticity]. Wydawnictwo Quaestio.

Ziółkowska, J. (2016). *Samobójstwo. Analiza narracji osób po próbach samobójczych* [Suicide. An analysis of suicide attempters' narratives]. PWN.

Ziółkowska, J., & Galasiński, D. (2017). Discursive construction of fatherly suicide. *Critical Discourse Studies*, *14*(2), 150–166. https://doi.org/10.1080/17405904.2016.1250650

# 2 Self in Suicide

## Introduction

In this chapter, we are primarily interested in institutional discourses of suicide. We want to examine how suicide is constructed in public (medical and activist) discourses and then contrast them with the stories of those who either killed themselves or attempted to do so. We are particularly interested in how a person taking their life is represented in public discourses; how they are represented as an actor deciding to end and/or ending their life.

Our main argument is that institutional discourses remove the person from their accounts of suicide. Suicide happens and is not done. The person taking their life is either only implied in the public accounts or, at best, relegated to doing things that are not directly related to taking their life. In contrast, stories of lived experiences show different relevancies where the nature of suicide is hidden, while the individual's agency is preserved. We point to this difference between the public and 'private' discourses and comment on its significance.

## Institutional Views of Suicide

Suicide is normally understood as the result of actions taken against the self by a person with the intention of ending their life. Such an understanding assumes the person's knowledge and awareness that the most likely consequence of their activities will be their death. While definitions and descriptions of suicide and suicidal behaviour are linked to several factors (Silverman, 2006), De Leo, Burgis, Bertolote, Kerkhof, and Bille-Brahe (2006) indicate the four elements contained in all the definitions of suicide analysed: (1) death is an outcome of the behaviour, (2) agency, (3) intent to die, and (4) awareness of the outcome of the act undertaken (see also: Farberow, 1980; Maris, Berman, & Silverman, 2000). Therefore, in suicidal behaviours, we have an actor independently deciding to take their

DOI: 10.4324/9781032672847-2

life; the individual is at the centre of the suicidal act, and it is their intent that leads to and defines suicide. As Andriessen (2006) writes, suicide is explicitly an individual decision and act (see also: Jaworski, 2010). Even if we assume that the time preceding the suicide attempt is associated with an altered state of consciousness (for example, close-mindedness and fixation on purpose, see: Shneidman, 1993; 1996; Baumeister, 1990), it is still accepted that the suicidal person is intentionally pursuing their death and is the agent in the suicidal act.

However, the progressive medicalisation of suicide and suicidal behaviour (Marsh, 2010) has resulted in the increased significance of terminology, classification, and standardised approaches thereto. Consequently, the first calls of the National Institute of Mental Health to unify the systems of classification of suicidal behaviour were made in the 1970s (Pokorny, 1974). And yet, despite almost 50 years of debate, a common unified terminology and classification of suicidal behaviour remains rather elusive (Silverman & De Leo, 2016; Goodfellow, Kõlves & de Leo, 2018). This is so, even though to understand, assess, predict, and act preventively against suicide, it is necessary to come up with a consistent system of understanding suicide and its types, as well as classifying various related behaviours (Silverman, 2006; also Leenaars et al., 1997; Rudd & Joiner, 1998; Shneidman, 1985).

In this chapter, we are primarily interested in the two sources of medical discourse for suicide. First, we examine the diagnostic manuals and their accounts of suicide. Then, we briefly discuss the dominant definitions of suicide.

### *Diagnostic Manuals*

There are two diagnostic manuals commonly used by the international mental health community: the recently introduced 11th iteration of the *International Classification of Mental and Behavioural Disorders* (ICD), prepared and published by the World Health Organisation (WHO) (2024) and the *Diagnostic and Statistical Manual of Mental Disorders* (DSM), prepared and published by the American Psychiatric Association (APA) (2022), currently in its text-revised fifth edition (DSM-5-TR).

The two documents operate at different levels. The ICD-11 is intended for a global audience, and as the 'ultimate' guideline for how to diagnose mental illness; on the other hand, the DSM is intended for American psychiatry. Both manuals are intended to offer a perspective-free classification of diseases.

As expected, there is much literature on the status, kinds, uses, and forms of classification of mental disorders. Evaluations of the two manuals range widely, from being pronounced as a conceptual framework for diagnosis (Bertelsen, 1999) and a major and helpful step for psychiatry (e.g., Owens, 2000; Jablensky, 1999), an agreed text based on current empirical data (Frances & Egger, 1999; Nathan & Langenbucher, 1999), to studies aiming to improve the classifications (e.g., Regier et al., 1998; Maj, 1998; Strain, 2005). Critics of the manuals' reliability (Kirk & Kutchins, 1994; also studies in Kirk, 2005) accuse them of creating diseases (Kutchins & Kirk, 1999; Parker et al., 1995).

There are two main lines of criticism levied at the diagnostic manuals. Both texts are charged with removing both the individual's experiences of distress as well as the social context in which the individual operates. For example, Phillips (2005) argues that clinical goals are in contradiction with those of the manuals (also Berganz, Mezzich, & Pouncey, 2005; Mezzich & Berganza, 2005); Gottschalk (2000) posits that if the current understating of self is in terms of changeability, the psychiatric classification prevents us actually from acknowledging it (also Corin, Rangaswami, & Padmavati, 2004). The other line of criticism challenges the classification's clarity. Parker (2004) argues that the guidelines are uninformative for clinical use and display a disturbing lack of rigour (also Pilgrim, 2007; Kirk & Hsieh, 2004).

Interestingly, suicide sits on the manuals' margins. Only the current version of the DSM attempts to offer advice on what constitutes suicidal behaviour; ICD-11 continues to see suicide in a very cursory way. However, they both do offer an interesting insight into how suicide is viewed in psychiatry, and this is why we would like to examine their discourses.

In our discussion, we focus on the 'canonical' English-language version of both manuals. However, there is a Polish translation of the DSM-5-TR; while the DSM is not intended for use in Poland, the translation suggests that it is relevant, for example, for researchers. We are interested in how the two language versions compare, guided by our earlier discovery that the English and Polish versions of the ICD-10 diagnostic criteria differ significantly (Galasinski, 2008).

## Suicide and the Self

In this section, we begin with an analysis of the text of the criteria for suicidal behaviour as stipulated in the DSM-5-TR. The current version, for the first time, proposes to consider suicidal behaviour a mental disorder in its own right. Up until the current, text-revised fifth edition, suicidal behaviour had been seen as only indicative of other mental illnesses (e.g., depression). The change proposed by the APA is a major move in the process of medicalising suicide.

These are the proposed criteria for suicidal behaviour disorder:

A. Within the last 24 months, the individual has made a suicide attempt. Note: A suicide attempt is a self-initiated sequence of behaviours by an individual who, at the time of initiation, expected that the set of actions would lead to his or her own death. (The 'time of initiation' is the time when a behavior took place that involved applying the method.)
B. The act does not meet the criteria for nonsuicidal self-injury—that is, it does not involve self-injury directed to the surface of the body undertaken to induce relief from a negative feeling/cognitive state or to achieve a positive mood state.
C. The diagnosis is not applied to suicidal ideation or to preparatory acts.
D. The act was not initiated during a state of delirium or confusion.
E. The act was not undertaken solely for a political or religious objective. (APA, 2022, p. 1683)

The criteria start by explicitly focusing on the individual. The sentence in criterion A is in active voice, underscoring the action taken by the individual. By using the verb *make*, which refers to a material process (Halliday, 1994), the text of the criterion emphasises agency behind the action. However, the reference to a generic 'suicide attempt' is likely to establish a nosological criterion rather than refer to meaningful action. Indeed, in the remaining criteria, the individual and their agency vanish.

In the note to criterion A, the focus changes to a 'self-initiated sequence of behaviours', with the agent replaced by the adverbial phrase ('by an individual'). Suicide is no longer something that an individual does, but it is simply a behaviour, an object rather than an action. Moreover, despite the phrase suggesting intent ('self-initiated'), the reference to behaviour introduces inconsistency, as the behaviour does not have to be intentional, planned, or agentive.

Perhaps surprisingly, the following sentence re-introduces agency to the individual but only in terms of mental activity. The individual behind the suicide attempt can only be said to expect something, rather than engage in an intentional action; indeed, expecting is the only action explicitly ascribed to the individual. The lack of clarity in the two sentences is underscored by the fact that the DSM speaks of actions again in the latter part of the sentence. However, while the individual's expectations are directed at the set of actions (earlier referred to as behaviours), the set itself has no owner, so to speak. It is constructed to lead to something as if being an independent object, without an agent behind it.

The confusion in the criteria continues in the sentence in parenthesis. Once again, the text refers to a behaviour that simply took place, rather than to an individual engaged in their action as an agent. The text of the criteria removes the person behind suicide and continues to construct suicide and suicide attempts as objects to inspect. It is worth pointing out that what was initially a set of behaviours, then a set of actions, becomes 'the act' in criteria D and E.

Interestingly, the backgrounding (i.e., removing from the explicit form of the sentence) of the person goes further. Criterion B implies human intervention through reference to the self, and yet, the person is immediately rendered in terms of their body and its surface, while the feelings and cognitive states do not have anyone having them. There is no one feeling the feelings in the text of the DSM; in fact, the feelings seem external to the person. This continues in criterion C where mental processes are referred to as 'suicidal ideation'. But, even more interestingly, what commonsensically seems to include a host of actions on the part of a person is reduced to mere 'preparatory acts'. What are they? What constitutes them, when they end, is not reflected upon.

However, such reflection seems important. If a person makes a noose, seconds before hanging themselves, is this still preparation or is it already suicidal behaviour? If they put the noose on their neck, is it still preparation or is it already an initiation of the 'behaviour'? Do you have to jump off the stool to stop the preparation? Such questions are important because they determine the nosological criteria of the potential diagnosis. This is especially important since the DSM later stipulated that after initiating a suicide attempt, an individual can change their mind or someone can intervene. The cut-off point when suicidal behaviour starts is of crucial importance, it seems.

We point to the confusion underpinning the text because it offers a significant insight into how institutional psychiatry sees suicide and the problems with the concept and the act. This can be seen both at the level of language and content of the text. The shifting between references to behaviour and actions is a good example of the conceptual confusion in the text. In terms of the content, if suicide and suicide attempt are defined through an individual's intent, then, surely stopping someone from ingesting the full amount of medication or poison is irrelevant as to whether an attempt has been made or not. And yet, the DSM gives this exact example as one for not making the diagnosis.

Moreover, we would argue that if the intent to commit suicide is crucial, it is also crucial to define suicidal behaviour through explicit reference to individuals as agents about to take their lives. References to a notional act or behaviour might only be useful in maintaining a medical narrative of objects to be inspected. Unfortunately, they lose the essence of suicidal action.

Let us now make a few comments on the Polish translation of the DSM-5-TR (APA, 2024). There are significant differences in how the criteria are rendered. Consider the first sentence of the description of a suicide attempt. The English text stipulates:

> A suicide attempt is a self-initiated sequence of behaviors by an individual.

Meanwhile, the translation of the Polish text into English is:

> A suicide attempt is a series of actions independently carried out by a person.[1]
>
> (APA, 2024, p. 1055)

The changes are significant. What in English is a behaviour, in Polish becomes an action. While the English text speaks only of initiating, referring only to the beginning of the behaviour, the Polish text speaks of 'carrying out', focusing on the entire process. Grammatically, the two sentences are also different; the phrase 'self-initiated' renders itself much more easily to become an attribute. Polish is not as malleable in word formation and so, the Polish text has an embedded clause ('independently carried out').

This sentence suggests a shift towards constructing agency in the Polish text of the DSM. This continues in the second sentence. The English text reads:

> The 'time of initiation' is the time when a behavior took place that involved applying the method.

On the other hand, the Polish text reads:

> The time of commencement is the time when the person begins the carrying out the adopted method.[2]
>
> (APA, 2024, p. 1055)

The Polish text changes the original, introducing a reference to an individual engaged in suicidal behaviour. This significantly changes the conceptualisation of suicidal behaviour, from apersonal to agentive. There are several possibilities as to why such changes might have been made. They range from a commonsensical understanding of suicide as involving action, through the dominant understanding of suicidal behaviour in Polish psychiatry, to attempting to render the Polish version in a text that will be considered well-written for the Polish reader. Regardless of the reasons, the changes, we think, are not only significant but also quite welcome. We believe that maintaining agency and subjectivity in institutional accounts of suicide is important and positive.

The removal of the suicidal self is consistent with how suicidal actions are also presented in the new edition of the ICD. Here are the relevant definitions from the ICD-11:

> Suicidal behaviour: Concrete actions, such as buying a gun or stockpiling medication, that are taken in preparation for fulfilling a wish to end one's life but that do not constitute an actual suicide attempt.
>
> Suicidal ideation: Thoughts, ideas, or ruminations about the possibility of ending one's life, ranging from thinking that one would be better off dead to formulation of elaborate plans.
>
> Suicide attempt: A specific episode of self-harming behaviour undertaken with the conscious intention of ending one's life.

All actions referred to in the texts are made into objects, starting with 'concrete actions', through 'buying', 'thoughts, ideas, or ruminations', 'self-harming behaviour' and 'ending'. These are all likely to be highly complex sets of actions carried out by individuals, and yet, the individuals are not even mentioned in the ICD-11 accounts.

Not only is there no individual doing the thinking or wishing in those accounts, but there is no single action rendered through verbs there. Suicide attempts or behaviour are all rendered through nominalisations.[3] No one thinks, behaves, acts, buys, or stockpiles; all those actions are transformed into objects ready for psychiatric inspection, whether clinical or research. Indeed, as has been observed many times (see, for example, Galasiński, 2008), rendering diagnostic criteria through contextless objects removes the individuals' unique experiences and presents them as universal and identifiable by psychiatry.

In this section, we explored the latest instances of how suicide is represented in medical discourses, focusing in particular on the construction of the self in such accounts. As was probably to be expected, the self is hardly present in the accounts of suicide. Suicide happens in such texts rather than someone doing it, performing it, or taking their life away, as the agent. This lack of agentivity is also reflected in the definitions of suicide beyond the diagnostic criteria. We briefly examine it in the next sections.

### *Definitions of Suicide*

The removal of the person and their agency from accounts of suicide can also be observed in definitions other than in the diagnostic manuals.[4] Most of the definitions we analysed were taken from earlier articles offering reviews and systematic reviews of definitions of suicide in suicidology (Silverman, 2006; De Leo et al., 2006; Goodfellow et al., 2018). In addition, we also made searches in suicidology's leading journals (*Suicide & Life-Threatening Behavior, Crisis, Death Studies,* and *Archives of Suicide Research*), and looked for articles in the MeDLINE database (via PubMed). In such a way, we compiled a list of 30 definitions used in suicidological literature, which we analysed. In this section, we briefly examine such definitions.

Consider a few examples:

**Extract 1**

A fatal wilful self-inflicted life-threatening act without an apparent desire to live.

(Davis, 1988)

**Extract 2**

an act inflicted upon oneself with the intention to kill oneself.

(Rosenberg et al., 1988)

**Extract 3**

a death that is caused by a self-inflicted intentional action or behavior.

(Silverman & Maris, 1995)

**Extract 4**

a self-inflicted act led to the person's death.

(Goldsmith et al., 2002)

**Extract 5**

Self-initiated, intentional death.

(Ivanoff, 1989)

**Extract 6**

Fatal self-inflicted, self-destructive act with explicit or inferred intent to die.

(Institute of Medicine, 2001)

The definitions are consistent in not defining suicide through what a person taking their life does. The individual's participation is implied through reference to either an unattributed action (e.g., 'self-inflicted act', 'self-induced annihilation') or mental state (e.g., 'intentional death', 'wilful act'). There are also no references to actions; the phrases implying human participation are used as attributes of acts or behaviours. The drive to remove the person linguistically can lead to definitions that, when taken at face value, are quite bizarre:

**Extract 7**

> All behaviour that seeks and finds the solution to an existential problem by making an attempt on the life of the subject.
>
> (Baechler, 1980)

Behaviours cannot seek anything, and they are also unlikely to have existential problems; behaviours also cannot make attempts on anyone's life. The definition shifts the agency from the person to an acontextual abstract object-behaviour, which is anthropomorphised in the text. Even more bizarrely, the agency structure of the sentence positions the behaviour as making an attempt on a person's life, making them a recipient of the behaviour's actions.

We also suggest that the function of the noun 'subject' in the definition is to depersonalise the individual and, in the process, suicide itself. The noun recontextualises a unique individual into an object of scientific, and perhaps also clinical, gaze. The definition is perhaps an excellent example of what has been known after Foucault (1973) as the 'medical gaze'. A person, with all their experiences and contexts, is reformulated into an object of scrutiny.

Expressions referring to mental states such as 'desire to live', 'intention to kill oneself', or 'intent to die' are also used as if they existed on their own without any person, token, or type actually holding them. Just as in the ICD, where complex experiences are rendered as unqualified nouns, for example, 'loss of interest' or 'indecisiveness' (see Galasiński, 2008), the definitions of suicide also refer to abstract 'mental symptoms', rather than to experiences of those who take their lives.

Notably, only mental states are referred to in the definitions. It is consistent with today's dominant constructions of suicide, which place it in the person (Marsh, 2010; Battin, 1995; Pridmore, 2011) and ignore the possibility of the person being in a social, economic, or political context that might have a significant impact upon the decision to kill themselves. This is despite the fact that suicidology is well aware of suicide occurring in certain social circumstances (governmental austerity measures, certain institutional contexts, for example, Branas et al., 2015; Flynn et al., 2017).

We would like to end this section quoting one last definition, from Shneidman, one of the founders of modern suicidology, who writes:

**Extract 8**

> Suicide is a conscious act of self-induced annihilation, best understood as a multi-dimensional malaise in a needful individual who defines an issue for which suicide is perceived as the best solution.
>
> (Shneidman, 1985)

Let us first point out a similarity between this definition and the proposed DSM diagnostic criteria. While in both accounts the individual is mentioned, they are only attributed mental actions. In the above definition, the individual is described as defining an issue, a process located somewhere on the borderline between mental and verbal. Indeed, as the individual is said only to define an issue, they are constructed as uninvolved in the suicide. Not only does suicide not have anyone who performs it, but the person who actually does it is constructed only as defining things.

We are not suggesting, of course, that anyone reading those definitions will have any difficulty in understanding that the individual is also the person who kills themselves. Our argument is not about text clarity; it is about the way the relationship between the act of suicide and the suicidal person is constructed. To our surprise, it is common not to construct a direct relationship between the person and the act of taking their life. Linguistically, the definitions obfuscate it and rely on the reader to supply a coherent reading of the definition and, through this, construct the relationship for themselves.

## Removing Agency

Before we move to juxtapose institutional discourses with narratives underpinned by lived experience, we would like to discuss one other aspect of public discourses on suicide. For some time now, both institutions and academics (for review see: Mishara & Dargis, 2019) have been asking people not to use the phrase 'commit suicide' and replace it with 'die by suicide' or 'die of suicide'.

In a recent article on perceptions of words and phrases referring to suicide and suicide behaviour, Padamanthan et al. (2019) attempt to engage with the much-discussed issue of how to speak of suicide in an evidence-based manner. It is the first study we know that attempts to give claims of evidential validity. Of the descriptors for suicide, 'took their own life' and 'died by suicide' received the highest median scores, while 'topped themselves' and 'successful suicide' received the lowest. Notably, the scores for 'committed suicide' were the most varied; only responses to this phrase covered the entire range. Those who had personal experience of suicide were more likely to find it acceptable than those whose experience of suicide was limited to work or volunteering.

Among the 274 participants who provided free-text comments, the most common reasons for choosing 'commit suicide' were accuracy and common usage, with some disputing its criminal connotations. Many people who had been personally affected by suicide referred to the clarity of the phrase, while those who had been affected by someone else's experience preferred it because it was direct and non-euphemistic (Padamanthan et al., 2019). A different approach to the study of suicide-related terms was taken by Parrott, Britt, Hayes, and Albright (2020) where they compiled a list of 98 suicide-related terms and phrases from a variety of sources (e.g., research literature, blogs, news sites, librarians, mental health professionals). Practising clinicians and members of the American Association of Suicidology (AAS) were asked to indicate whether they considered each term valid or invalid. Interestingly, the phrase 'die by/of suicide' was not listed, while 'commit suicide' was seen as validated by 84% of respondents (62 out of 74) (Parrott et al., 2020).

So far, the discussion of such language had been based on assumptions about, and predominantly referred to the meaning of the word 'commit'. It is argued both in academic discourse (Mishara & Dargis, 2019; Sommer-Rotenberg, 1998; Sinyor et al., 2018; Nielsen et al., 2016, Nielsen, n.d.) and more widely in activist contexts (Olson, 2011; Caruso, n.d.) that the use of the phrase 'commit suicide' places suicide firmly in the legal, criminalised domain. The claim is based on the well-rehearsed arguments that suicide is stigmatising and stigmatised (Sudak et al., 2008; Carpiniello & Pinna, 2017). Using a phrase that might be regarded as suggesting criminality can be argued to add to the stigmatisation of suicide (Mindhacks, 2017; Beaton et al., 2013). This is why the phrase is removed from the lexicon of responsible reporting on suicide; more widely, institutions advise against using it. Indeed, the text of the DSM-5-TR already incorporates the phrase 'die of suicide'.

Before we continue, it is perhaps worth mentioning that claims that the verb 'commit' makes what it refers to illegal or sinful are fallacious. Indeed, we could argue that proponents of such claims commit fallacies, which are neither illegal nor sinful. You can as easily commit an act of bravery, an act of love, kindness, or courage, none of which are even negative.

This possibility of the verb 'commit' entering phrases with negative and positive connotations (though, admittedly, the former are more common) results from the fact that 'commit' in such phrases can be seen as a 'light' verb. This is to say that the verb carries little or no meaning at all in a phrase. Its meaning is bestowed on it by the noun it forms a phrase with (Butt, 2003; Grimshaw & Mester, 1988). And so, in phrases such as 'take a break' or 'make a request', the verbs are largely irrelevant. One could argue, of course, how light the verb 'commit' is (Nenonen et al., 2017), still the arguments based on its meaning should be made with some caution.

Our view is that any language policy must be based on solid empirical evidence. There are two aspects of such evidence that seem pertinent. First, Padamanthan and co-authors (2019) suggest that it is for people with personal experience of suicide that the phrase 'commit suicide' is more acceptable. Given this, we do not believe we have a right to judge or police how people who experienced a great personal tragedy should refer to it. Second, the evidence that 'commit suicide' is problematic and contributes to the stigma of suicide is still ambivalent at the very best.

To date, a study by Howell and co-authors (2023) shows that the phrase 'committed suicide' is perceived as more applicable to a suicide portrayed as immoral than to a suicide portrayed neutrally. As they argue, judgements of the applicability of 'committed suicide' statements vary systematically as a function of how a death by suicide is depicted. They continue to argue, however, that this might have to do with the perception of intentionality carried by the phrase. Kollareth and co-authors (2019) argue that the phrase 'commit suicide' is perceived as agentive, and, therefore refers to the high intentionality of the action, regardless of the moral undertones.

This is, indeed, the crucial point in the discussion on the use of the phrase 'commit suicide'. It is replaced by a phrase that removes the person's agency in taking their own life. 'Die by suicide' suggests that death happens, much like in any illness. And yet, suicide is not like any illness at all. The person does something to 'die by suicide'. The suggested phrase changes the way we are encouraged to see suicide. It is no longer an action of a person who takes their life, but an event that happens to them. In a nutshell, the proposed change in language also removes the intentional aspect of suicide.

## Agency in Lived Experience

In this section, we seek to juxtapose constructions of the self and the self's agency in the public discourses discussed above with how they are constructed in 'private' narratives. We are interested in examining the extent to which institutional discourses match the relevancies of discourses narrating the lived experiences of suicide. In this case, we offer two sets of extracts. We start with how the self is narrated in the suicide notes and then move to extracts from our interviews.

We argue that there are significant differences in how suicide is constructed in the two discourses. While public/institutional discourses focus on removing the individual's responsibility and agency, in contrast, individuals writing suicide notes or speaking about their suicide attempt stress their agency. While institutions choose to stress the nature of the act, calling it suicide, the stories of life experiences attempt to hide the fact that what the individual did was suicide (for an extended discussion of euphemising suicide, see Galasiński, 2017).

Consider first a few fragments of suicide notes:

**Extract 9**

I apologise to all in my family, friends. I know you will not forgive me for this act.

I am sorry.

**Extract 10**

Forgive me, dear girls, for my disgraceful act, but I cannot differently, I cannot put it off anymore, because in the end I would not have the strength to do what I want to do.

**Extract 11**

I am sorry for I have done. I have always loved you [addressing many] and I do.

**Extract 12**

I am not asking for forgiveness. What I am about to do cannot be forgiven.

**Extract 13**

I am taking this horrific step to free you all from the evil I spread around.

The notes refer to their authors' suicides, yet none explicitly uses the word 'suicide'. 'Suicide' is replaced by nouns such as 'act' or 'step', or simply with reference to what was done. The removal of the word 'suicide' is particularly interesting because the references sometimes do carry value judgements. In Extracts 11 and 13, the authors speak of a 'disgraceful act',[5] and a 'horrific step'; Extract 12 seems to up the ante by referring to something that cannot be forgiven. Such evaluations of 'the act' are consistently negative in our dataset and yet, they do not refer to suicide directly.

Significantly, while suicide is hidden from the explicit narrative, responsibility for it is acknowledged in all five extracts, and linguistic agency is preserved in the latter three (Extracts 11–13). Such agency, however, is even more explicitly constructed in notes that do not make references to ‘an act’. Consider:

**Extract 14**

I am departing. It is hard for me. Forgive.

**Extract 15**

Dear children. I am departing.

I am terribly sorry.

**Extract 16**

I have departed of my own accord.

**Extract 17**

I have decided to leave this life. I apologise to you [addressing many].

All four extracts construct the individual as an agent in the act. The agency is strengthened by the use of the verb *odchodzić* (or *odejść*—which is its perfective form), ‘to depart’ or ‘to leave’ (with a connotation of walking). The primary meaning of the verb positions it as referring to a material process—and it is material processes that are the primary vehicle of rendering action, with the performer of the action explicitly rendered as an agent.

In other meanings, the verb is used to refer to the unilateral breaking up of relationships and as a euphemistic reference to dying. The use of the verb as referring to suicide is marked, as out of the ordinary, thereby introducing ambiguity as to what exactly is referred to. In other words, the letters in 14–16 could very well be written as farewell letters written by people who died of an illness or simply broke up a relationship. Once again, while an individual’s agency is preserved, reference to suicide is at the very least, ambiguous.

Interestingly, similar narratives can be observed in the interview dataset.

**Extract 18**

I quit my studies, where I had always been a top-grade student. I did not tell my parents I had quit the studies. And after two years they started

> suspecting that something was very wrong. And I simply knew that I had to tell them. And I decided that this was a better solution than facing all that. But as I say, I never planned it, it was just one moment. I simply went to the park for a walk and did it.

**Extract 19**

> I had a lot of problems which all built up and that is why I wanted to do what I wanted.

**Extract 20**

> Over the week before I had had various thoughts [...] and it was building up. I had depression and more and more suicidal thoughts were coming to my mind, like exactly to finish with all this. I could not sleep at night and I was worried about my family [unclear] and in the end I decided to take this step and I do not know whether I regret it now.

Judging by the extracts, mentioning suicide explicitly is very difficult. The three interviewees go out of their way, it seems, to not do it, offering a range of ways in which to only imply their suicide attempt. What is crucial, however, from our point of view, is that all three construct themselves as responsible for their actions.

We realise that in Extracts 19 and 20 the agency is linguistically mediated by reference to mental processes (such as wanting or deciding), but there is no doubt that it is implied. Moreover, much like in suicide letters, our interviewees were explicit in constructing agency for them when using verbs that were not immediately associated with suicide. Thus, our interviewees talked about jumping or cutting, thereby taking a position of agency in such narratives. It is only suicide itself that seems unmentionable.

We see such avoidances as resulting from the stigma associated with suicide (Frey et al., 2016). Suicide is one of the most stigmatising acts, and although there is evidence that today's stigma is subtler (Feigelman et al., 2009), people who died in an act of suicide are still regarded as blameworthy, weak, cowardly, selfish, and sinful in comparison to those who died, for example, through cancer (Sand et al., 2013). Consequently, those who survive the suicidal death of a loved one not only have to cope with the loss but may also have to face negative attitudes and comments about the deceased (Evans & Abrahamson, 2020). Some studies show that survivors of suicide can be blamed for the act (Gibbons, 2024; Loy & Boelk, 2014). As Feigelman and co-authors (2009) argue, such stigmatisation of suicidal death can exacerbate survivors' grief difficulties and mental health problems, with children suffering from negative outcomes (Cerel & Aldrich, 2011; Ratnarajah & Schofield, 2011).

What is interesting for us here is that public and private discourses perceive stigma differently. When narrating their experiences, those who were about to kill themselves and those who made a serious attempt on their lives avoid labelling their actions in terms of suicide. However, in institutional discourses, suicide is consistently mentioned explicitly. It seems that institutional discourses do exactly the opposite of what they set out to do. Moreover, while institutional discourses want to construct suicide as non-agentive, those engaging in suicidal behaviour do exactly the opposite.

## Conclusion

This chapter examined public discourses of suicide, focusing primarily on how it is constructed in the diagnostic manuals. We have argued that suicide is represented as an objective event rather than an action taken by an individual. The individual is consistently backgrounded in psychiatric accounts of suicide. Human participation in suicide is, at best, implied. The manuals' constructions of suicide and the individual committing it are consistent in their definitions of the act. Invariably, the definitions of suicide represent it as without explicit action of an individual. The same argument can be made about activist discourses advocating a particular way of speaking about suicide.

We then contrasted such representations with how suicide is represented in narratives, either in suicide notes or in interviews after a serious suicide attempt. Such 'private' representations are very different from those in institutional discourses. The key difference is that, while institutional discourses remove the individual and their agency, such agency is explicitly maintained in the lived experience narratives. Time and again, both authors of suicide notes and our interviewees stressed their agency and responsibility in their suicide act. However, consistently they backgrounded the nature of the act. Suicide was regularly euphemised into more generic acts or events. In our conclusions, we would like to offer some commentary on our findings.

In a popular article, the sociologist Julie Phillips (2019) argues that taboos around suicide are loosening and it has become more available socially. Indeed, accepting suicide as a solution for an incurable disease or even getting tired of life is rising (Phillips & Luth, 2020). Phillips and Luth (2020) argue that the efforts to reduce the stigma around suicide may have had some unwanted effects. If suicide is not as negative as we thought, perhaps it is more acceptable. It is worth noting that research by Oliffe and co-authors (2011; 2012) suggests that stigma can be seen as protective in the case of men who do not want to inflict pain on their close ones.

We propose that constructions of suicide without reference to the individual and their agency may well be part of discourses contributing to suicide's acceptability. Representing suicide as an event only happening to people frames it more as an accident and can be summarised with the well-trodden and colloquial phrase 'bad things happen', or its more popular vulgar equivalent. However well-meaning the assumptions behind phrases such as 'die by suicide' may be, if they contribute to the social and psychological availability of suicide, they must be re-examined. We accept, nevertheless, that more research is needed between the stigma, representations of suicide, and its acceptability.

We also think that the differences in constructions of the self in suicide between institutional and 'private' discourses raise important issues. The first is that they create a gap between how institutions and people with lived experiences of suicide construct themselves and their actions. The significant mismatch between what is relevant for medicine and the person is likely to lead to rejection of the public message and, possibly, to difficulties in clinical encounters.

Finally, and perhaps more importantly, removing agency from how suicide is conceptualised moves it closer to a deterministic view. Things just happen and if no one is agentive in what happens, there is perhaps also nothing anyone can do to stop it. We suggest that such a representation of suicide misses an important dimension in both preventative and clinical work. Agency in suicide must not be seen only as agency in committing the act. Agency in suicide must also mean the agency to not do it. In other words, by removing agency from suicide, an opportunity to turn the agency around is also removed.

Therefore, we argue for the inclusion of agency in suicide for two reasons. First, because this is how our informants constructed themselves in their accounts of their suicide or suicide attempts—that is, in both suicide contexts we studied. Second, we call for constructing suicide agentively because such constructions would be consistent with constructions of not committing suicide. If a person is an unfettered agent taking their life, we suggest they are also an unfettered person staying alive.

This discussion is continued in the next chapter where we move to consider accounts of lived experiences of suicide. We start our discussion by examining constructions of agency with reference to the individual engaged in suicidal action. However, we are also interested in the agency around suicide, and what the person does when they are not engaging in taking their life. We are interested in the margins of suicide and explore waiting for one's death as part of the suicide act.

## Notes

1 Here is the original text in Polish: *Próba samobójcza to samodzielnie przeprowadzony ciąg działań przez osobę...*
2 Here is the original text in Polish: *'Czas ich rozpoczynania' to ten czas, kiedy osoba przystępuje do realizacji obranej metody.*
3 Actions, doing things, are normally rendered with the use of verbs. Nominalisation changes this and replaces verbs with nouns, turning acting into actions. And so, rather than saying that an individual thinks about suicide, the same process is rendered as an object through nouns such as thoughts.
4 The argument is based on a more extended discussion of suicide definitions that we offered in Galasiński and Ziółkowska (2020).
5 This is how we translate the Polish word *postępek* used by the writer, as it carries negative connotations, possibly of transgression, possibly a crime.

## References

American Psychiatric Association [APA] (2022). *Diagnostic and Statistical Manual of Mental Disorders, Fifth Edition, Text Revision (DSM-5-TR)*. American Psychiatric Association Publishing.

American Psychiatric Association [APA] (2024). *Kryteria Diagnostyczne Zaburzeń Psychicznych DSM-5-TR*. Edra Urban & Partner (Original work published 2022).

Andriessen, K. (2006). On 'intention' in the definition of suicide. *Suicide & Life-Threatening Behavior*, 36(5), 533–538. https://doi.org/10.1521/suli.2006.36.5.533

Baechler, J. (1980). A strategic theory. *Suicide and Life-Threatening Behavior, 10*(2), 70–99.

Battin, M. P. (1995). *Ethical issues in suicide*. Prentice-Hall, Inc.

Baumeister, R. F. (1990). Suicide as escape from self. *Psychological Review*, *97*(1), 90–113. https://doi.org/10.1037/0033-295X.97.1.90

Beaton, S., Forster, P., & Maple, M. (2013). Suicide and language: Why we shouldn't use the 'C' word. *InPsych*, *35*(1), 30–31.

Berganza, C. E., Mezzich, J. E., & Pouncey, C. (2005). Concepts of disease. *Psychopathology*, *38*(4), 166–170. https://doi.org/10.1159/000086084

Bertelsen, A. (1999). Reflections on the clinical utility of the ICD-10 and DSM-IV classifications and their diagnostic criteria. *Australian and New Zealand Journal of Psychiatry*, *33*(22), 166–173. https://doi.org/10.1046/j.1440-1614.1999.00525.x

Branas, C. C., Kastanaki, A. E., Michalodimitrakis, M., Tzougas, J., Kranioti, E. F., Theodorakis, P. N., Carr, B. G., & Wiebe, D. J. (2015). The impact of economic austerity and prosperity events on suicide in Greece. *BMJ Open*, *5*, e005619. https://doi.org/10.1136/bmjopen-2014-005619

Butt, M. (2003). The light verb jungle. In G. Aygen, C. Bowern, & C. Quinn (Eds.), *Harvard Working Papers in Linguistics 9* (pp. 1–49). GSAS/Dudley House Workshop on Light Verbs.

Carpiniello, B., & Pinna, F. (2017). The reciprocal relationship between suicidality and stigma. *Frontiers in Psychiatry*, *8*, 35. https://doi.org/10.3389/fpsyt.2017.00035

Caruso, K. (n.d.). *Stop saying 'committed suicide'. Say 'died by suicide' instead.* Suicide.org. www.suicide.org/stop-saying-committed-suicide.html

Cerel, J., & Aldrich, R. S. (2011). The impact of suicide on children and adolescents. In J. R. Jordan & J. L. McIntosh (Eds.), *Grief after suicide* (pp. 81–92). Routledge.

Corin, E., Rangaswami, T., & Padmavati, R. (2004). Living through a staggering world: The play of signifiers in early psychosis in South India. In J. H. Jenkins & R. J. Barrett (Eds.), *Schizophrenia, culture, and subjectivity* (pp. 110–145). Cambridge University Press.

Davis, J. H. (1988). Suicidal investigation and classification of death by coroners and medical examiners. In J. Nolan (Ed.), *The suicide case: Investigation and trial of insurance claims. Tort and insurance practice section* (pp. 33–50). The American Bar Association.

De Leo, D., Burgis, S., Bertolote, J. M., Kerkhof, A. J., & Bille-Brahe, U. (2006). Definitions of suicidal behavior: Lessons learned from the WHO/EURO Multicentre Study. *Crisis*, *27*(1), 4–15. https://doi.org/10.1027/0227-5910.27.1.4

Evans, A., & Abrahamson, K. (2020). The influence of stigma on suicide bereavement: A systematic review. *Journal of Psychosocial Nursing and Mental Health Services*, *58*(4), 21–27. https://doi.org/10.3928/02793695-20200127-02

Farberow, N. L. (Ed.). (1980). *The many faces of suicide: Indirect self-destructive behavior*. McGraw-Hill Book Company.

Feigelman, W., Gorman, B. S., & Jordan, J. R. (2009). Stigmatization and suicide bereavement. *Death Studies*, *33*(7), 591–608. https://doi.org/10.1080/07481180902979973

Flynn, S., Nyathi, T., Tham, S. G., Williams, A., Windfuhr, K., Kapur, N., Appleby, L., & Shaw, J. (2017). Suicide by mental health in-patients under observation. *Psychological Medicine*, *47*(13), 2238–2245. https://doi.org/10.1017/S0033291717000630

Foucault, M. (1973). *The birth of the clinic: An archaeology of medical perception*. Tavistock Publications Limited.

Frances, A. J., & Egger, H. L. (1999). Whither psychiatric diagnosis. *Australian and New Zealand Journal of Psychiatry*, *33*(2), 161–165. https://doi.org/10.1046/j.1440-1614.1999.00534.x

Frey, L. M., Hans, J. D., & Cerel, J. (2016). Perceptions of suicide stigma. *Crisis*, *37*(2), 95–103. https://doi.org/10.1027/0227-5910/a000358

Galasiński, D. (2008). *Men's discourses of depression*. Palgrave Macmillan.

Galasiński, D. (2017). *Discourses of men's suicide notes: A qualitative analysis*. Bloomsbury Publishing.

Galasiński, D., & Ziółkowska, J. (2020). A moment outside time: A critical discourse analytic perspective on dominant constructions of suicide. In Z. Demjen (Ed.), *Applying linguistics in illness and healthcare contexts* (pp. 349–371). Bloomsbury.

Gibbons, R. (2024). Someone is to blame: The impact of suicide on the mind of the bereaved (including clinicians). *BJPsych Bulletin*, 1–5. https://doi.org/10.1192/bjb.2024.37
Goldsmith, S. K., Pellmar, T. C., Kleinman, A. M., & Bunney, W. E. (Eds.). (2002). *Reducing suicide: A national imperative*. National Academies Press.
Goodfellow, B., Kõlves, K., & De Leo, D. (2018). Contemporary nomenclatures of suicidal behaviors: A systematic literature review. *Suicide and Life-Threatening Behavior*, *48*(3), 353–366. https://doi.org/10.1111/sltb.12354
Gottschalk, S. (2000). Escape from insanity. 'Mental disorder' in the postmodern moment. In D. Fee (Ed.), *Pathology and the postmodern: Mental illness as discourse and experience* (pp. 18–48). Sage.
Grimshaw, J., & Mester, A. (1988). Light verbs and Θ-marking. *Linguistic Inquiry* *19*(2), 205–232.
Halliday, M. A. K. (1994). *An introduction to functional grammar* (2nd ed.). Edward Arnold.
Howell, A. J., Mack, E. C., Scavuzzo, R. R., & Tomaras, C. A. (2023). Effects of context on perceptions of the language of suicide. *Advances in Mental Health*, *21*(2), 165–178. https://doi.org/10.1080/18387357.2023.2169179
Institute of Medicine [IOM] (2001). *Health and behavior: The interplay of biological, behavioral, and societal influences*. National Academy Press.
Ivanoff, A. (1989). Identifying psychological correlates of suicidal behavior in jail and detention facilities. *Psychiatric Quarterly*, *60*(1), 73–84. https://doi.org/10.1007/BF01064364
Jablensky, A. (1999). The nature of psychiatric classification. *Australian and New Zealand Journal of Psychiatry*, *33*(2), 137–144. https://doi.org/10.1046/j.1440-1614.1999.00535.x
Jaworski, K. (2010). The author, agency and suicide. *Social Identities*, *16*(5), 675–687. https://doi.org/10.1080/13504630.2010.509572
Kirk, S. A. (2005). *Mental disorders*. Columbia University Press.
Kirk, S. A., & Hsieh, D. K. (2004). Diagnostic consistency in assessing conduct disorder. *American Journal of Orthopsychiatry*, *74*(1), 43–55. https://doi.org/10.1037/0002-9432.74.1.43
Kirk, S. A., & Kutchins, H. (1994). The myth of reliability of DSM. *Journal of Mind and Behavior, 15*(1–2), 71–86.
Kollareth, D., Allam, A., & Russell, J. A. (2019). On judging the immorality of someone having taken his or her own life. *Social Cognition, 37*(6), 547–570. https://doi.org/10.1521/soco.2019.37.6.547
Kutchins, H., & Kirk, S. A. (1999). *Making us crazy*. Constable.
Leenaars, A. A., De Leo, D., Diekstra, R. F., Goldney, R. D., Kelleher, M. J., Lester, D., & Nordstrom, P. (1997). Consultations for research in suicidology. *Archives of Suicide Research*, *3*(2), 139–151. https://doi.org/10.1023/A:1009695021180
Loy, M., & Boelk, A. (2014). *Losing a parent to suicide. Using lived experiences to inform bereavement counseling*. Routledge.
Maj, M. (1998). Critique of the DSM-IV operational diagnostic criteria for schizophrenia. *British Journal of Psychiatry*, 172(6), 458–460. https://doi.org/10.1192/bjp.172.6.458.

Maris, R. W., Berman, A. L., & Silverman, M. M. (2000). *Comprehensive textbook of suicidology*. The Guilford Press.

Marsh, I. (2010). *Suicide: Foucault, history and truth*. Cambridge University Press.

Mezzich, J. E., & Berganza, C. E. (2005). Purposes and models of diagnostic systems. *Psychopathology, 38*(4), 162–165. https://doi.org/10.1159/000086083

Mindhacks. (2017). Should we stop saying 'commit' suicide? https://mindhacks.com/2017/08/12/should-we-stop-saying-commit-suicide/#comment-476868

Mishara, B. L., & Dargis, L. (2019). Systematic comparison of recommendations for safe messaging about suicide in public communications. *Journal of Affective Disorders, 244*, 124–154. https://doi.org/10.1016/j.jad.2018.09.031

Nathan, P. E., & Langenbucher, J. W. (1999). Psychopathology: Description and classification. *Annual Review of Psychology, 50*, 79–107. https://doi.org/10.1146/annurev.psych.50.1.79

Nenonen, M., Mulli, J., Nikolaev, A., & Penttilä, E. (2017). How light can a light verb be? Predication patterns in V + NP constructions in English, Finnish, German and Russian. In M. Luodonpää-Manni, E. Penttilä, & J. Viimaranta (Eds.), *Empirical approaches to cognitive linguistics: Analyzing real-life data* (pp. 75–106). Cambridge Scholars Publishing.

Nielsen, E. (n.d.). *Mind your 'C's and 'S's: The language of self-harm and suicide (and why it matters)*. IMH Blog. https://imhblog.wordpress.com/2016/01/22/emma-nielsen-mind-your-cs-and-ss-the-language-of-self-harm-and-suicide-and-why-it-matters/

Nielsen, E., Padmanathan, P., & Knipe, D. (2016). Commit* to change? A call to end the publication of the phrase 'commit* suicide'. *Wellcome Open Research, 1*, 21. https://doi.org/10.12688/wellcomeopenres.10333.1

Oliffe, J. L., Han, C. S., Ogrodniczuk, J. S., Phillips, J. C., & Roy, P. (2011). Suicide from the perspectives of older men who experience depression: A gender analysis. *American Journal of Men's Health, 5*(5), 444–454. https://doi.org/10.1177/1557988311408410

Oliffe, J. L., Ogrodniczuk, J. S., Bottorff, J. L., Johnson, J. L., & Hoyak, K. (2012). 'You feel like you can't live anymore': Suicide from the perspectives of Canadian men who experience depression. *Social Science & Medicine, 74*(4), 506–514. https://doi.org/10.1016/j.socscimed.2010.03.057

Olson, R. (2011). *Suicide and language*. Centre for Suicide Prevention. www.suicideinfo.ca/resource/suicideandlanguage/

Owens, D. G. C. (2000). The challenges of diagnosis and continuing patient assessment. *International Journal of Psychiatry in Clinical Practice, 4*(1), 13–18. https://doi.org/10.1080/13651500050518488

Padmanathan, P., Biddle, L., Hall, K., Scowcroft, E., Nielsen, E., & Knipe, D. (2019). Language use and suicide: An online cross-sectional survey. *PloS One, 14*(6), e0217473. https://doi.org/10.1371/journal.pone.0217473

Parker, G. (2004). Critique of the guidelines for the treatment of depression. *Australian and New Zealand Journal of Psychiatry, 38*(11–12), 885–890. https://doi.org/10.1080/j.1440-1614.2004.01479.x

Parker, I., Georgaca, E., Harper, D., McLaughlin, T., & Stowell-Smith, M. (1995). *Deconstructing psychopathology*. Sage.

Parrott, S., Britt, B. C., Hayes, J. L., & Albright, D. L. (2020). Social media and suicide: A validation of terms to help identify suicide-related social media posts. *Journal of Evidence-Based Social Work*, *17*(5), 624–634. https://doi.org/10.1080/26408066.2020.1788478

Phillips, J. (2005). Idiographic formulations, symbols, narratives, context and meaning. *Psychopathology*, *38*(4), 180–184. https://doi.org/10.1159/000086087

Phillips, J. (2019). *The dangerous shifting cultural narratives around suicide*. The Straits Times. www.straitstimes.com/opinion/the-dangerous-shifting-cultural-narratives-around-suicide

Phillips, J. A., & Luth, E. A. (2020). Beliefs about suicide acceptability in the United States: How do they affect suicide mortality? *The Journals of Gerontology: Series B, Psychological Sciences and Social Sciences*, *75*(2), 414–425. https://doi.org/10.1093/geronb/gbx153

Pilgrim, D. (2007). The survival of psychiatric diagnosis. *Social Science & Medicine, 65*(3), 536–547. https://doi.org/10.1016/j.socscimed.2007.03.054

Pokorny, A. D. (1974). A scheme for classifying suicidal behaviors. In A. T. Beck, H. L. P. Resnik, & D. J. Lettieri (Eds.), *The prediction of suicide* (pp. 29–44). Charles Press.

Pridmore, S. (2011). Medicalisation of suicide. *The Malaysian Journal of Medical Sciences*, *18*(4), 78–83.

Ratnarajah, D., & Schofield, M. J. (2007). Parental suicide and its aftermath: A review. *Journal of Family Studies*, *13*(1), 78–93. https://doi.org/10.5172/jfs.327.13.1.78

Regier, D. A., Kaelber, C. T., Rae, D. S., Farmer, M. E., Knauper, B., Kessler, R. C., & Norquist, G. S. (1998). Limitations of diagnostic criteria and assessment instruments for mental disorders. *Archives of General Psychiatry*, *55*(2), 109–115. https://doi.org/10.1001/archpsyc.55.2.109

Rosenberg, M. L., Davidson, L. E., Smith, J. C., Berman, A. L., Buzbee, H., Gantner, G., Gay, G. A., Moore-Lewis, B., Millis D. H., & Murray, D. (1988). Operational criteria for the determination of suicide. *Journal of Forensic Sciences*, *33*(6), 1445–1456.

Rudd, M. D., & Joiner, T. (1998). The assessment management and treatment of suicidality: Toward clinically informed and balanced standards of care. *Clinical Psychology: Science and Practice*, *5*(2), 135–150. https://doi.org/10.1111/j.1468-2850.1998.tb00140.x

Sand, E., Gordon, K. H., & Bresin, K. (2013). The impact of specifying suicide as the cause of death in an obituary. *Crisis*, *43*(1), 63–66. https://doi.org/10.1027/0227-5910/a000154

Shneidman, E. S. (1985). *Definition of suicide*. John Wiley & Sons.

Shneidman, E. S. (1993). *Suicide as psychache: A clinical approach to self-destructive behavior*. Jason Aronson, Inc.

Shneidman, E. S. (1996). *The suicidal mind*. Oxford University Press.

Silverman, M. M. (2006). The language of suicidology. *Suicide and Life-Threatening Behavior*, *36*(5), 519–532. https://doi.org/10.1521/suli.2006.36.5.519
Silverman, M. M., & De Leo, D. (2016). Why there is a need for an international nomenclature and classification system for suicide. *Crisis*, *37*(2), 83–87. https://doi.org/10.1027/0227-5910/a000419
Silverman, M. M., & Maris, R. W. (1995). The prevention of suicidal behaviors: An overview. *Suicide and Life-Threatening Behavior*, *25*(1), 10–21.
Sinyor, M., Schaffer, A., Heisel, M. J., Picard, A., Adamson, G., Cheung, C. P., Katz, L. Y., Jetly, R., & Sareen, J. (2018). Media guidelines for reporting on suicide: 2017 update of the Canadian Psychiatric Association Policy Paper. *Canadian Journal of Psychiatry. Revue canadienne de psychiatrie*, *63*(3), 182–196. https://doi.org/10.1177/0706743717753147
Sommer-Rotenberg, D. (1998). Suicide and language. *CMAJ: Canadian Medical Association Journal*, *159*(3), 239–240.
Strain, J. J. (2005). Psychiatric diagnostic dilemmas in the medical setting. *Australian and New Zealand Journal of Psychiatry*, *39*(9), 764–771. https://doi.org/10.1080/j.1440-1614.2005.01681.x
Sudak, H., Maxim, K., & Carpenter, M. (2008). Suicide and stigma: A review of the literature and personal reflections. *Academic Psychiatry: The Journal of the American Association of Directors of Psychiatric Residency Training and the Association for Academic Psychiatry*, *32*(2), 136–142. https://doi.org/10.1176/appi.ap.32.2.136
World Health Organisation [WHO]. (2024). *International Classification of Mental and Behavioural Disorders 11th Revision*. Retrieved from: https://icd.who.int/en

## Appendix

**Extract 9**

PRZEPRASZAM WSZYSTKICH MOICH Z RODZINY, ZNAJOMYCH WIEM ŻE NIE WYBACZYCIE MI ZA TEN CZYN... PRZEPRASZAM

**Extract 10**

Wybaczcie mi kochane dziewczyny mój haniebny postępek ale nie mogę inaczej nie mogę nie dłużej zwlekać bo w końcu nie miałbym siły wykonać co zamierzam.

**Extract 11**

Przepraszam za to co zrobiłem zawsze Was bardzo kochałem i kocham.

**Extract 12**

Nie proszę Cię o wybaczenie, tego co zamierzam zrobić wybaczyć nie można.

**Extract 13**

Robię ten straszny krok aby uwolnić Was wszystkich od zła które rozsiewam wokół.

**Extract 14**

Odchodzę. Ciężko mi. Wybacz.

**Extract 15**

Kochane dzieci odchodzę

jest mi ogromnie przykro

**Extract 16**

Odszedłem z własnej woli.

**Extract 17**

Postanowiłem odejść z tego życia Przepraszam was.

**Extract 18**

I: [...] rzuciłam studia. gdzie: zawsze byłam piątkową uczennicą. y: i: i też rodzicom nie powiedziałam że rzuciłam te studia. no i w końcu po tych dwóch latach zaczęli podejrzewać że coś jest coś jest grubo nie tak. (.) e: i po prostu no m: tak no wiedziałam że muszę im o tym powiedzieć. (.) i (stwierdziłam) że to jest lepsze wyjście niż niż niż niż stawienie stawienie temu wszystkiemu czoła po prostu. ale mówię nie planowałam tego to po prostu było tak w: jednej chwili. po prostu poszłam na spacer do parku i (..) i tam to zrobiłam.

**Extract 19**

I: [...]miałem swoje problemy i to się skumulowało i dlatego. (.) no. chciałem zrobić to co chciałem. (.)

Extract 20

I: […] już tydzień wcześniej takie miałem różne myśli (znaczy po prostu w tych dniach) to się nawarstwiało miałem depresję i i coraz częściej przychodziły mi takie myśli samobójcze właśnie jak żeby po prostu zakończyć z tym wszystkim. (..) nie mogłem spać po nocach i: (..) [wzdycha] bałem się o swoją rodzinę też bo wiadomo że że dziecko (niejasne) w końcu [wzdycha] zdecydowałem się na ten krok no i nie wiem teraz (czy to) żałuję tego

# 3 Self and Agency

## Introduction

In the previous chapter, we focused on institutional discourses of suicide and juxtaposed them with narratives of individuals who wrote suicide notes before taking their lives or who provided accounts of their serious suicide attempts after the event. We argued that the two discourses are underpinned by different relevancies. Institutional discourses focus on removing the individual's agency in the suicidal act while, at the same time, maintaining the nature of the act as explicit. The discourse of lived experiences of suicide did the opposite. While maintaining responsibility and agency behind the act, it backgrounded its suicidality. This, we argued, might have significant consequences in suicide prevention as well as clinical work.

In this chapter, we examine constructions of agency with reference to the individual engaged in suicidal action. Agency is a definitional feature of suicide. It is the acting individual who is at the centre of the suicidal act, and it is their intent that leads to suicide. We are interested in the stories of what those who are about to take their lives do when engaged in suicide action. We want to extend our argument that understanding suicide only as a person's death is unhelpful, as most definitions of suicide propose (Galasiński & Ziółkowska, 2020a).

We want to see how agency is constructed both in relation to suicide and to the individual's actions in the period surrounding the suicidal act. This builds upon our earlier work on the suicidal process and the agency within it (Galasiński & Ziółkowska, 2020b). We also want to explore the narratives of all those actions that are seemingly on the margins of suicide, particularly those accounts that describe waiting for suicide and death as part of the process of taking one's own life.

DOI: 10.4324/9781032672847-3

### *Agency in Suicide*

Suicide is the result of actions taken by a person against themselves with the intention of ending their life. This presupposes the knowledge and awareness that the most likely consequence of one's actions will be death. Even if we assume that the time preceding the suicide attempt is associated with an altered state of consciousness (see, for example, Shneidman, 1993; 1996; Baumeister, 1990), it is still accepted that the suicidal person is intentionally pursuing suicide and is the agent of the suicidal act.

Yet, suicidologists pay little attention to agency, despite it being a fundamental component of suicide. Webb (2011) argues that the understanding of suicidal experiences and behaviours must go far beyond the determination of the strength of association between variables and the comparison of statistics of suicide deaths. Lester and Stack (2015) (also Hjelmeland, 2016; Bantjes & Swartz, 2019; 2020) reinforce this message by stating that the mere correlation of different variables does not bring suicidology closer to understanding suicide. This, in our view, must include significant research effort into understanding the agency of the individual undertaking a suicidal act.

Some interest in agency and suicide can be seen in the critical strand of suicidology (White, 2017; Chandler et al., 2022). Two anthropologists, Broz and Münster (2015), recognise agency as fundamental to the concept of suicide. However, they also point to the notion of victimhood or 'patiency' in suicide, where the suicidal act is seen as influenced by external forces such as demons, kinship, illness, or violence. For them, this tension between agency and patiency is the essence of suicide. Agency also relates to the concepts of intentionality and responsibility. They argue that while suicide requires a singular and undivided intention, cultural aetiologies rarely assign full responsibility to the individual. This creates a tension in suicide discourse between singular intention and diffused responsibility, mediated by sociological and psychological approaches (Broz & Münster, 2015). Indeed, as we argued in the previous chapter, today's institutional accounts of suicide do not encourage examination of agency, thus making it irrelevant to how suicide is conceptualised.

Following Marsh (2010; 2013), Broz and Münster (2015) see psychology, psychiatry, and their cognates (Rose, 1988) as diminishing the agency-as-responsibility of the suicidal individual by framing suicide as caused by mental illness or psychological problems. Thus, suicidal individuals are seen as mentally ill and not fully responsible for their actions (see Marsh, 2013). Such pathologising frames suicide as indicative of a medical condition rather than a personal agency, suggesting external causes similar to sociological factors. This is supported by constructions of suicide as an event with a backgrounded role of the individual.

In this chapter we want to problematise agency and go beyond suicidal intention. We argue that the constructed agency in narratives becomes more complex than what one could assume based on the intentionality of suicidal behaviour. This is because agency does not only apply to the act of taking one's life; agency is also constructed in stories seemingly marginal to suicide. What happens in the time before death is as pertinent to describing the process of suicide as is the physical attempt on one's life. We also want to explore the linguistic picture of agency in narratives off the centre of the suicidal process. Our objective is to demonstrate that agency is a dynamic characteristic of narratives about suicidal experiences, subject to change in the context of telling the story. Crucially, we want to show the complexity of suicide.

Therefore, we are interested in how individuals who write or speak about their suicide or suicide attempt position themselves in terms of linguistic agency. We aim to understand how 'doing things' is represented in discourse. Our focus lies on the lexicogrammatical form, rather than on the contents of what was written. In other words, it was more important to us whether the linguistic form rendered the 'doer' as doing things.

## Waiting

We would like to start this section with two suicide letters constructing a stereotypical suicide:

> **Extract 1**
>
> I didn't go to school today. I decided to commit suicide. I tried to cut my veins, but I was not very successful. I overdosed on [medication] and I am waiting for what will happen. I have done it because I do not want to go to school. Otherwise, I would have to go tomorrow, and I would not bear it.

> **Extract 2**
>
> I have been taking bad decisions. The decision about my death was conscious and well-thought-out. No one has talked me into death. I am solely responsible for the death through exsanguination.

There is no doubt or hesitation in the text; both notes explicitly ascribe agency to their authors. In Extract 1, agency is rendered canonically. Verbs are in active voice, predicated on the speaker who is positioned as the subject of the clauses. In Extract 2, agency is constructed more indirectly through nominalisations.[1] However, any potential doubts that could be raised by such phrasing are dispelled with the statement ascribing responsibility to the author of the note.

Now, we propose the two extracts as stereotypically rendering suicide because they construct it as self-inflicted. The agency is unquestionable, and the focus of the two extracts is almost entirely on the outcome. In contrast, however, many suicide letters suggest a much more complicated route to suicide and death. The agency is considerably less clear, and the process is not a straight line between physical self-harm and death. Consider first the following three suicide notes:

**Extract 3**

Tell me – what am I to do so that you would want to be with me? You don't want to see me – so you said – so, I cannot come over. But I am waiting for the opportunity. Never in my life have I expected such words from you, so this is why it is such a blow for me. Unsurvivable. I could have expected everything but not what happened to me. All the time I have worked so you could be comfortable. There are various moments in life but this low, after so many years, something one could not have thought about.

**Extract 4**

It is hard to come to terms with that the woman one loves wants another man and despises her past love and does not appreciate the efforts one makes for her. But I will bear it all so that you are happy. I am staying in [city name] so that I can gather my thoughts and fulfil your wish but I am waiting for a sign from you so that I could come home. You have crushed me so I am no longer myself. I am putting an appearance for people but I do not know how long I can keep it up. I know nothing but I agree to everything, as long as you could be mine and love me again.

**Extract 5**

I am still deceiving myself that something which will stop me will happen. There is still a spark of hope left, to be sure, a fleeting one, but still. Perhaps someone will ask me why here, in this place. The reason is simple. I do not want anyone to interrupt me and here it will almost certainly not happen.

All three extracts refer to a period of waiting before taking suicidal action, and significantly, the waiting is constructed in active terms, with the author taking an active role in the wait. However, there is also a tension implied in the extracts. The active waiting is counterbalanced by the actions (or their absence) and wishes of the external agent, the addressee of the letter, particularly in Extract 5. The author of the note explicitly represents his waiting as dependent on the actions of another. The wait can stop if the hope comes true.

The other aspect of these notes is the complexity of agency they introduce. Crucially, the notes do not undermine the agency in killing oneself; they introduce complexity on the margins of the act. It is the waiting that becomes the pivot around which suicidal action turns and from which it stems.

Extracts 3 and 4 construct a similar picture. Both construct a broken man; the author of the note, who had been crushed and lost himself. He is ready to give in, but for keeping the relationship with the note addressee. The notes also set up a counterbalance to the broken man—the waiting. Both men seem to offer a choice between life and death. Suicide becomes something that is caused by another while it is also an act taken by the decision of the writing person. Nothing seems straightforward as the note authors' subjectivities depend as much on another person as they depend on themselves. This is perhaps best seen in Extract 5, where the explicit wait for someone to stop the suicide is juxtaposed with the explicit wish not to be interrupted.

Consider now another group of extracts in which the writers construct themselves as actively waiting:

**Extract 6**

I keep writing some more, because I want to persuade you that life and health are beautiful until one has them.

**Extract 7**

It's [exact time]. From one moment to another I can see that my life makes no sense. I have talked to [first name] a moment ago and she has depressed me even more. She said nothing, but I mean the tone of her voice. It was so unhappy as if she had wanted to say I am so unhappy with you.

**Extract 8**

Right. Dear sister, end of feeling sorry for myself and I am sorry that I turn to you the most, but I had to talk to someone.

In Extract 6, the writer constructs himself as going back to writing, as if not wanting to finish; writing seems to keep him from taking his life. The note is described as having the aim to persuade and is thereby constructed as important and having to be written carefully. As a result, we see the note author as engaged in an activity before his suicidal death, taking the time to get the note right.

Yet, it is the reference to writing, we suggest, that constructs the 'true' agency; this is where the author is in full control. Similarly, in Extract 7, the author represents himself as pondering life and realising things. In addition, he writes about a conversation with another person, also positioning himself as the agent in the conversation. The expression 'from one moment to another' not only suggests the passing of time but also underscores the repetitive nature of the activity. The same can be said of the reference to the end in Chapter 8.

So far, we have discussed notes in which waiting is limited to the period shortly before the person takes their life. The accounts can be assumed to convey the time in which the suicide process had already started; the waiting only makes it last a bit longer. In the next two extracts, the waiting is considerably longer. Consider:

**Extract 9**

Today it is Tuesday, [date], and I am performing it tomorrow, that is [date] because today I still need to attend to a matter.

**Extract 10**

I have finally managed to hang the dog-lead. I will go for a walk the day after tomorrow and I am going to my death.

The notes offer a record of a process that takes days. The authors write about a considerable amount of time in which they need to put off taking their lives, which, to make it clear, they eventually did. Both notes indicate that events were put in motion, but there were tasks to be completed before the suicidal death. Indeed, in Extract 10, the hanging of the dog-lead describes the scene of the suicidal act waiting for the note author to be ready. Significantly, in both notes, the authors are positioned as actors or doers, fully in control of the situation. They decide to put the act off. The agency of the person waiting to end their life cannot be made more explicit.

To finish this discussion, we would like to discuss one last group of suicide letters that are in contrast to those above. Consider:

**Extract 11**

You killed. You killed. You killed. You killed.

**Extract 12**

[First name] you know what it is like when you cannot cope with what I now think, I want you [first name]. I would forgive you anything. I wanted you to hold me, how I miss it.

You cheated on me. Why?

Why did you kill me?

There are at least two layers of agency here. There is the physical reality in which the authors of the notes killed themselves. However, there is also the reality constructed in the notes. Suicide is positioned as resulting from a loved one's actions. The note in Extract 11, quoted in its entirety, leaves no doubt as to who is responsible for the suicidal death of the note author.

Our argument here is that while agency behind suicide is represented as complex and ambivalent, the notes represent waiting for suicide as being in control of the person taking their life. In most accounts of waiting, the note authors' actions are unfettered; there are no external agents that have an impact on what the authors do. It is waiting, considering or feeling sorry for oneself that allows the authors to position themselves as unfettered agents. Such accounts of waiting raise significant issues in understanding the suicide process. We shall take them up later on in the conclusions.

## Agency of Not Killing Oneself

In the previous section, we discussed constructions of waiting as an agentive action of those about to take their life. We argued that such agency could be seen as having a significant part in the suicidal process. This section continues the discussion, focusing on the accounts of the suicidal process narrated after a suicide attempt. We are interested in the extent to which informants' narratives ex-post facto mirror representations of the person as having control over the time preceding the suicidal act.

Consider the following extracts:

**Extract 13**

I: How long did you prepare yourself for suicide?
A: I mean, I delayed it, as much as possible, in time.

**Extract 14**

Well, then I didn't want to kill myself, perhaps sometimes. No, no, I kind of wanted a bit. But on the other hand, I rejected it. Because on balance I didn't want to. I wouldn't like to hurt her.

**Extract 15** (**the informant describes attempting to drown**)

And as I put one foot in the water, I went back. [...] I thought I would wait a while. I went to the children, to my son and daughter-in-law. In the meantime, as I was drinking coffee, my husband arrived. He felt something, that I am not OK but he did not know that I was thinking about something like suicide.

In all three extracts, the informants construct themselves in agentive terms in the period before suicide. The delay in Extract 13 is mirrored in Extract 14, where the informant describes rejecting the wish to kill himself. Interestingly, in the extract, it is the wish to commit suicide that is undermined by the hedge 'kind of', while rejection is presented in fully agentive terms.

We pick up the long account of the informant's unfulfilled attempt to drown at the moment when she puts her foot in the water. At this point, there is a shift in the narrative and the informant introduces the second part, which begins with a decision to wait. The informant constructs herself as actively thinking (deciding) about suicide. She continues with an account of her subsequent actions, unburdened by what happened minutes earlier (unquoted here).

What is significant in such accounts is that agency is not only attributed to the decision to take one's life or the physical action. Crucially, these extracts also demonstrate agency in not killing oneself. There are accounts in which the interviewees talk about rejecting a course of action, taking time to think or to wait.

Some interviewees explicitly described their wishes or decisions that had been kept in check by their agency:

**Extract 16**

I do not know whether I took the decision now or then. It is quite blurred. Because at any time I can change my mind, so I do not know whether the decision is taken at the moment.

**Extract 17**

I started thinking that perhaps it is a good idea to do it, execute it, and there will be peace. Everything will end. But later I stopped thinking about it. It came back later and the last moment that pushed me to do it was news that someone did not do something in time that they promised to do.

In Extract 16, the informant explicitly positions himself as capable of revoking his decisions, leading to the ambivalence of when a decision is made. His agency is mediated by reference to his capacity. Although it can be argued that such a reference constructs agency as weaker, the interviewee still shows himself as in control over what happens. In Extract 17, stopping to think about suicide is conveyed in fully agentive terms. While initiating and stopping thoughts of suicide presents the speaker as in control, subsequently describing the thoughts as 'coming back' presents as if they were outside the thinking actor. Not taking the last step after stopping to think about it seems the only part of the suicide attempt that the informant is in control of.

We realise, of course, that the story leads to a suicide attempt. Our argument here, however, is that while suicide, as portrayed in suicide letters, is often constructed as something over which people have no control, our analysis shows that the stories we analyse do suggest control. We believe this can lead to a rethinking of prevention methods.

The waiting we have just discussed was narrated in stories concerning decisions about whether to take one's life. Significantly, it was also referred to when our informants talked about the suicidal process in the situation of suicide underway. Consider:

**Extract 18**

So, I went into the bathtub, ran the water and I was standing and thinking whether I was doing the right thing. I was thinking and thinking about telling my husband, perhaps he would have stopped me. But I say, no, I must try. Perhaps it will work now. If not now, it will never work for me.

**Extract 19**

I made myself breakfast but I could not eat anything. I was waiting for my mother to wake up so that she could take care of [the child]. And so, when my little son went to her room, I went to the bathroom, locked it, and took the scalpel and I was standing with it. I was ready for it and cut my veins.

**Extract 20**

I panicked [...]. I thought I will not wait till the evening because if my dad tells his brother, they will take me to hospital the same day. So, I took the double-edge scalpel.

There are explicit references to both waiting and thinking in the extracts above. All convey the time before the suicidal act. What is significant in such references is that they represent the speaking person as in control of the situation. Extract 19 shows waiting as strategic. The speaking person, a mother, took the time to wait for her mother to wake up. The account is explicitly agentive, and the speaker offers reasons for her actions. The informant's actions are considered and well-thought-out. Extract 20 is different; the control that is conveyed here is that of stopping the wait.

In the three extracts above, the control rendered concerns both the waiting and the suicidal action. The narratives are calm, and collected, and there is no emotional crisis conveyed. Everything is in hand. In particular, Extract 19 shows both control and awareness of the person's surroundings. This is not always the case, and we would like to end with two final extracts that offer some complexity to the picture. Consider:

**Extract 21**

> It's not like a person stands on a bridge and flies off. It is an internal struggle. At least with me, it was like that a split second decides about your life, that you will push yourself off and you fly down and it's the end of your life. It is the end. Because when you slowly prepare yourself and so on, doubts come. And if you want it, when you have decided, like me recently, then simply you go and suddenly you press away from the bridge and you go down. I did it like that and it was a struggle. And on the bridge, I didn't succeed.

This is an account of a planned attempt to jump off a bridge that did not happen. It is also a story of an internal struggle that didn't go away. However, it is also a story of the time before the jump. The internal struggle and the doubts are represented as external to the speaker. The phrase 'doubts come' presents internal struggle as an object rather than a process of thinking.

In contrast, the time before the jump is represented in active clauses with the person in the agentive position. This is crucial for our discussion here. Even though the time before suicide is represented in terms of ambivalence, there is a shift from ambivalence to action and the period before the jump is represented in active terms. We realise, of course, that in Extract 21 agency before the jump is presented as preparation. We propose, however, that the grammatical form is more important and, crucially, aligns with the pattern we describe in this chapter.

The final extract we want to discuss here is different.

**Extract 22**

> At the beginning of [month], a break with my girlfriend started. My parents went away and left me on my own at home. And basically, I cut myself off because I was sitting at home and felt like doing nothing. On the last day, I simply jumped into the noose on a sort of bar which I had attached to the wall and put a belt on it. I was hanging in the air and I do not know the last compunction, made me live. So, I grabbed the bed with my toes and took the noose off. I cried till the morning.

There is no intentional waiting here; the informant talks about 'hanging', a verb used without implying agency. What is significant, however, is that the informant constructs the time between the action and his death as an opportunity to stop the process.

In this section, we discussed the time before a suicidal action. There were two such constructions. First, our informants talked about the time from a medium- or long-term perspective. In other words, they talked about either waiting or delaying the engagement with suicide. Second, the time-scale was much shorter since the waiting time referred to was positioned within the suicidal action.

The most significant aspect of the data we collected is that the time before or within a suicidal attempt is constructed as under the control of the participant. There is no drama, or crisis referred; instead, there is a decision to defer or wait. This is significant because such data are mostly referred to in terms of ambivalence. We suggest that a more useful way to approach such times is by discussing agency. We take this up in our concluding remarks.

## Contesting Oneself

The previous section showed the ambivalent nature of suicidal agency. Consistently, it is only waiting, and not taking one's life that is constructed in agentive terms. The agency behind suicide is more complex. Therefore, this section aims to continue this discussion. Our focus here is on stories where the suicidal person's agency is taken away altogether. This is done in two ways. First, the interviewees explicitly undermine their decisions and actions by representing them as accidental or thoughtless. Second, the informants position themselves and their actions in relation to their close ones whose presence impacts their decisions.

### *Non-Agents*

Interview accounts of suicide attempts consistently showed suicide as something happening rather than stemming from a rational, thoughtful action. Agency is undermined while control over the suicide attempt is located outside the person. Put differently, suicide is constructed as an event rather than an intentional deed. Consider the most explicit account below:

**Extract 23**

> A: It all started because I did not take my pills for some time and so, I hanged myself. It is because of the pills, because I did not take them.

The story explicitly positions control over the suicidal act outside the speaker. The second part of the fragment positions the pills as the cause of what the interviewee did. While the subsequent clause introduces some ambivalence, the agency is primarily ascribed to the action of not taking pills rather than to suicide. In a way, the suicide attempt is constructed as outside the interviewee's control. Consider now some other accounts.

**Extract 24**

> As it happens, I do not know why I did it. I do not know. It was like a bit like a performance. I recorded myself swallowing those sixty pills of Clonazepam, two milligrams and an empty vodka bottle, a half litre and I put it on my Facebook.

**Extract 25**

> I do not know why I did it. I felt so lonely, I do not know. Lonely or something. I had everything at home. I wanted to cut my veins.

**Extract 26**

> And the last attempt [...], perhaps I am a serial suicide or something. Or perhaps it means that I am a loser or that I have some other motives, like a need for attention or crying for help or some such things. [...] but on the whole, I do not know my motives.

All three fragments undermine the attempt as a rational well-thought-out action. The interviewees show themselves as not knowing why they engaged in a suicide act. All three go further though. In Extract 24, the interviewee recasts the suicide attempt as a performance, as if the attempt was not real. Indeed, in contrast to the description of the suicide action, the account of the performance, including the references to recording and posting on social media, is presented in agentive terms. In Extract 25, the interviewee starts by presenting himself as not knowing why he tried to kill himself and juxtaposes it with 'having everything at home'. We read this as setting up a context in which the suicide attempt was unjustified.

Extract 26 is different; the interviewee uses references to his nature as a means of undermining the agency behind attempting to take his life. This leads to the reference of not knowing his motives; there is no agency in the extract. Instead, the picture is static with a description of the interviewee, which is passed as responsible for the suicide attempt.

The extracts above construct the interviewees as unable to understand what happened to them and what was going on in their heads. Consider two fragments in which the interviewees explicitly reject their thinking about suicide:

**Extract 27**

After lunch I started something, I deluded myself that I would do it. Suddenly. When I was coming out on leave (from hospital) I was not thinking about it. It did not cross my mind.

**Extract 28**

It was very stupid what I had done. I do not know. These terrible voices egged me on to doing that. I get a pill for sleeping and before sleeping, just before falling asleep they come to me and talk me into it all the time. But I do not want to listen to them and I reject them but despite that, I do come. I do not know where it comes from in my head. Does it turn over in my own head?

The interviewee's erroneous and misguided thinking (rendered by the verb *uroić*, 'to delude' (oneself)) is presented as contrary to her previous state of mind when she did not have suicidal thoughts. A similar verb is used in Extract 28. We translated *roić* as 'turn over in one's head' to stress the iterativity of the action. However, the verb carries the connotations of unwelcome and untrue thinking.

## Conclusion

In this chapter we discussed constructions of individuals' agency when engaged in suicidal action. We were interested in how suicidal action is represented and the actions in the time around the suicidal act. Both suicide letters and interviews showed that it was the time before suicidal action that was in the individual's full control. While the agency behind suicide is presented as complex and ambivalent, the waiting, considering, and feeling is where the agency of the individual engaged in suicidal action is presented as unfettered.

Our data and analyses pose questions on how mainstream research addresses issues of suicidal ambivalence. For suicidologists, ambivalence is the co-occurrence of two competing wishes: the wish to die (WTD) and the wish to live (WTL), and it has been of interest to suicidologists since the 1960s (Stengel, 1964; Kovacs & Beck, 1977; Brown et al., 2005; Bryan, 2020). Since Kovacs and Beck's (1977) study on the internal struggle during a suicide attempt, the methodology of ambivalence research has changed, and suicidologists now use more advanced methods of data collection and analysis. Cross-sectional designs are complemented by longitudinal ones and, more recently, the method of Ecological Momentary Assessment (EMA), which provides nuanced data collected in real time (see Kleiman et al., 2023). Researchers found that the discrepancy between an individual's WTL and WTD are risk factors for suicide risk (Brown et al., 2005; see also Harris et al., 2010; O'Connor et al., 2012). Bryan and co-authors (2016) have also shown that WTD and WTL ebb and flow dynamically throughout the treatment for suicidal thoughts and behaviours. Goods and co-authors (2020) and Oakey-Frost and co-authors (2023) have additionally demonstrated the importance of WTL as a protective factor against suicide. These studies suggest that WTL has the potential to 'destabilise' an individual's desire to die, acting as a stable trait-like quality with minimal variability.

Despite advances in methods of data analysis and increased efforts to collect sophisticated datasets, locating ambivalence in the context of progression from suicidal ideation to suicidal action remains largely unexplored (Bryan & Rudd, 2016). We have not found any answer to the question of whether ambivalence accompanies the person throughout the entire suicidal process, that is, from the suicidal ideation until the moment of the act (Harris et al., 2010). Early studies linked ambivalence to the act of suicide; Shneidman wrote: 'People who actually commit suicide are ambivalent about life and death at the moment they commit suicide' (Shneidman, 1998, p. 133). Similarly, Kovacs and Beck's (1977) study also referred to people's memories at the time of the suicidal act. Given the challenges of studying the progression from suicidal ideation to action, ambivalence is currently studied using prospective designs among individuals with a history of suicidal behaviour (e.g., Bryan et al., 2016; Goods et al., 2020; Oakey-Frost et al., 2023). While such a research model allows for the exploration of the dynamics of ambivalence, the question about the location of ambivalence in the context of progression from ideation to action is also a valid one.

Our data pose two questions. The first question centres on the source of the claims about ambivalence. Suicidologists tend to focus exclusively on the contents of what is written or said by the individual engaged in suicidal action. The problem for us, however, is that any discourse, written or spoken, cannot be seen only in terms of its content. Contents are rendered by particular linguistic forms. The arguments we make in this chapter are predominantly based on the language form of what was written or said. We do not propose, however, that our data offer better evidence or a truer perspective on suicidal agency. Rather, we suggest that they should be considered as offering a different perspective and that both perspectives must be considered.

Moreover, such arguments raise again the importance of qualitative discourse analysis in understanding suicide. By focusing on lived experience, that is to say, narratives rendering the experiential perspective of an individual engaged in suicidal action, we offer insight into the individual drama of suicide. We continue to believe that the dominant top-down methodological perspective of suicidology can and should be contrasted with the bottom-up perspective of discourse analysis. It is only in this way we can reach a fuller picture of suicide.

The second question posed by our analyses comes from the very focus of our chapter. Suicidological research commonly focuses on suicidal action. Moreover, it sees suicide in terms of its outcome: death. As such, suicidology loses sight of the fact that suicide is not simply a point in time in which a person dies. Not only does suicide take time, but dying itself takes time. Indeed, it is time where much can happen.

Such a time was perhaps first suggested in the Golden Gate studies, which focused on people who survived a jump off the Golden Gate Bridge in San Francisco, a very well-known suicide spot. One of the studies reports that people, admittedly with a strong intent to end their lives as judged by their actions, were not so sure during the fall down to the surface of the water (Rosen, 1975). Our previous study on the process of suicide (Galasiński & Ziółkowska, 2020) also shows how complex the time of ending one's own life is.

This is why we wanted to focus on the agency behind actions that are on the margins of suicide and under the radar of suicidology. What they show, again, is the complexity of suicide and suicide action. By focusing on such data, we stress the importance of viewing suicide not as an outcome, but as a multi-faceted process with multiple dimensions. Each of these dimensions contributes to the complexity of suicide, which can be used to focus on its prevention. The physical act of taking one's life is only one part of the overall process of suicide.

Our analyses offer at least one additional perspective. Suicidology commonly assumes the dramatism of suicide. Suicidologists speak of tunnel vision (e.g., Jesiolowski & Rogers, 2013; Shneidman, 1993), whereby the suicidal individual is incapable of seeing other perspectives and is drawn to suicidal action. Suicide is also assumed to be aimed at ending the unbearable psychic pain. Shneidman (1985) proposed that unbearable mental pain or 'psychache' is the central element in understanding suicide and suicidal behaviour. Suicide occurs when a person can no longer tolerate it. Shneidman (1985) and Orbach (2003) associate intolerable mental pain with a perceived lack of capacity to be loved, maintain control, protect one's self-image, avoid shame, and feel secure. These perceptions are often accompanied by a cluster of negative feelings including guilt, shame, defeat, humiliation, grief, rage, and a profound lack of hope for the future.

In our earlier work, we posed questions of such an understanding of suicide. Men's suicide notes consistently represented suicide as rational and well-thought-out (Galasiński, 2017). Ziółkowska's study (2016), in turn, shows that there is a sudden disappearance of any references to emotionality in the narratives referring to the time immediately before suicide. Both studies underscore the importance of narrative/textual evidence in understanding suicide.

Our study here supports our earlier findings. Consistently, we saw accounts where suicide was preceded by a period of consideration and waiting during which the suicidal individual had full control. Such stories were an interesting reflection of folk wisdom encouraging careful deliberation when making a decision. These stories present suicide as well-considered.

We already pointed to one significant consequence of such data for suicidology. Suicide must not be seen as boiling down to the physical extermination of life. The suicide process is significantly more complex. The second consequence is the problematisation of the assumption of the emotionality of suicide.

We realise, of course, that being in control of the process before taking one's life does not exclude the existence of emotional states that are difficult to bear. It does exclude, however, the notions of a universal tunnel vision where nothing else is considered or able to be considered. Our data show that individuals are in control of their lives. This, in our view, requires at least some change to how we conceptualise suicide.

In the next chapter, we continue exploring the subjectivities surrounding suicide, focusing specifically on its romanticisation. We explore the narratives that portray suicide as leading to actions or events that can be considered desirable or beautiful. In these accounts, the person who takes their life is positioned as a recipient of those actions or is at the centre of the events.

## Note

1 Nominalisation is the rendering of an action through a noun. And so, the action of kissing could be phrased as 'I kissed' or as 'my kiss'. The latter phrase is a case of nominalisation.

## References

Bantjes, J., & Swartz, L. (2019). 'What can we learn from first-person narratives?' The case of nonfatal suicidal behavior. *Qualitative Health Research*, *29*(10), 1497–1507. https://doi.org/10.1177/1049732319832869

Bantjes, J., & Swartz, L. (2020). The benefits of robust debate about the place of qualitative research in suicide prevention. *Qualitative Health Research*, *30*(6), 944–946. https://doi.org/10.1177/1049732320909104

Baumeister, R. F. (1990). Suicide as escape from self. *Psychological Review*, *97*(1), 90–113. https://doi.org/10.1037/0033-295X.97.1.90

Brown, G. K., Steer, R. A., Henriques, G. R., & Beck, A. T. (2005). The internal struggle between the wish to die and the wish to live: A risk factor for suicide. *American Journal of Psychiatry*, *162(*10), 1977–1999. https://doi.org/10.1176/appi.ajp.162.10.1977

Broz, L., & Münster, D. (2015). The anthropology of suicide: Ethnography and the tension of agency. In L. Broz & D. Münster (Eds.), *Suicide and agency* (pp. 3–24). Routledge.

Bryan, C. J. (2020). The temporal dynamics of the wish to live and the wish to die among suicidal individuals. In. A. C. Page & W. G. K. Stritzke (Eds.), *Alternatives to suicide. Beyond risk and toward a life worth living* (pp. 71–88). Academic Press.

Bryan, C. J., & Rudd, M. D. (2016). The importance of temporal dynamics in the transition from suicidal thought to behavior. *Clinical Psychology: Science and Practice*, *23*(1), 21–25. https://doi.org/10.1111/cpsp.12135

Bryan, C. J., Rudd, M. D., Peterson, A. L., Young-McCaughan, S., & Wertenberger, E. G. (2016). The ebb and flow of the wish to live and the wish to die among suicidal military personnel. *Journal of Affective Disorders*, *202*, 58–66. https://doi.org/10.1016/j.jad.2016.05.049

Chandler, A., Cover, R., & Fitzpatrick, S. J. (2022). Critical suicide studies, between methodology and ethics: Introduction. *Health*, *26*(1), 3–9. https://doi.org/10.1177/13634593211061

Galasiński, D. (2017). *Discourses of men's suicide notes: A qualitative analysis*. Bloomsbury.

Galasiński, D., & Ziółkowska, J. (2020a). A moment outside time: A critical discourse analytic perspective on dominant constructions of suicide. In Z. Demjen (Ed.), *Applying linguistics in illness and healthcare contexts* (pp. 349–371). Bloomsbury.

Galasiński, D., & Ziółkowska, J. (2020b). *Discursive constructions of the suicidal process*. Bloomsbury.

Goods, N. A., Page, A. C., Stritzke, W. G., Kyron, M. J., & Hooke, G. R. (2020). Daily monitoring of the wish to live and the wish to die with suicidal inpatients. In A. C. Page & W. G. K. Stritzke (Eds.), *Alternatives to suicide. Beyond risk and toward a life worth living* (pp. 89–110). Academic Press.
Harris, K. M., Mclean, J. P., Sheffield, J., & Jobes, D. (2010). The internal suicide debate hypothesis: Exploring the life versus death struggle. *Suicide and Life-Threatening Behavior, 40*(2), 181–92. https://doi.org/10.1016/j.comppsych.2011.09.007
Hjelmeland, H. (2016). A critical look at current suicide research. In J. White, I. Marsh, M. Kral, & J. Morris (Eds.), *Critical suicidology. Transforming suicide research and prevention for the 21st century* (pp. 31–55). UBC Press.
Jesiolowski, B. S., & Rogers, J. R. (2013). The phenomenology of suicide. In D. Lester & J. R. Rogers (Eds.), *Suicide: A global issue* (pp. 31–54). Praeger.
Kleiman, E. M., Glenn, C. R., & Liu, R. T. (2023). The use of advanced technology and statistical methods to predict and prevent suicide. *Nature Reviews Psychology, 2*(6), 347–359. https://doi.org/10.1038/s44159-023-00175-y
Kovacs, M., & Beck, A. T. (1977). The wish to die and the wish to live in attempted suicides. *Journal of Clinical Psychology, 33*(2), 361–365. https://doi.org/10.1002/1097-4679(197704)33:2<361::AID-JCLP2270330207>3.0.CO;2-H
Lester, D., & Stack, S. (2015). Conclusions. In D. Lester & S. Stack (Eds.), *Suicide as a dramatic performance* (pp. 323–331). Transaction Publishers.
Marsh, I. (2010). *Suicide: Foucault, history and truth*. Cambridge University Press.
Marsh, I. (2013). The uses of history in the unmaking of modern suicide. *Journal of Social History, 46*(3), 744–756. https://doi.org/10.1093/jsh/shs130
O'Connor, S. S., Jobes, D. A., Yeargin, M. K., FitzGerald, M. E., Rodríguez, V. M., Conrad, A. K., & Lineberry, T. W. (2012). A cross-sectional investigation of the suicidal spectrum: Typologies of suicidality based on ambivalence about living and dying. *Comprehensive Psychiatry, 53*(5), 461–467. https://doi.org/10.1016/j.comppsych.2011.09.007
Oakey-Frost, N., Moscardini, E. H., Cowan, T., Cohen, A., & Tucker, R. P. (2023). The temporal dynamics of wish to live, wish to die, and their short-term prospective relationships with suicidal desire. *Behavior Therapy, 54*(3), 584–594. https://doi.org/10.1016/j.beth.2022.12.011
Orbach, I. (2003). Mental pain and suicide. *Israel Journal of Psychiatry and Related Sciences, 40*(3), 191–201.
Rose, N. (1998). *Inventing our selves: Psychology, power, and personhood*. Cambridge University Press.
Rosen, D. H. (1975). Suicide survivors: A follow-up study of persons who survived jumping from the Golden Gate and San Francisco–Oakland Bay Bridges. *Western Journal of Medicine, 122*(4), 289–294.
Shneidman, E. S. (1985). *Definition of suicide*. John Wiley.
Shneidman, E. S. (1993). *Suicide as psychache: A clinical approach to self-destructive behavior*. Jason Aronson, Inc.
Shneidman, E. S. (1996). *The suicidal mind*. Oxford University Press.
Shneidman, E. S. (1998). *The suicidal mind*. Oxford University Press.
Stengel, E. (1964). *Suicide and attempted suicide*. Penguin Books.

Webb, D. (2011). *Thinking about suicide. Contemplating and comprehending the urge to die.* PCCS Books.
White, J. (2017). What can critical suicidology do? *Death Studies, 41*(8), 472–480. https://doi.org/10.1080/07481187.2017.1332901
Ziółkowska, J. (2016). *Samobójstwo. Analiza narracji osób po próbach samobójczych* [Suicide. An analysis of suicide attempters' narratives]. PWN.

## Appendix

### Extract 1

Nie poszłam więc dzisiaj do szkoły. Postanowiłam popełnić samobójstwo. Próbowałam podciąć sobie żyły ale nie bardzo mi to wyszło. Przedawkowałam jakiś lek chyba naproxen i czekam na to co będzie. Zrobiłam to ponieważ nie chcę nigdy więcej iść do szkoły. W przeciwnym razie musiałabym iść jutro a tego bym nie zniosła.

### Extract 2

Podejmowałem złe decyzje.

Decyzja o śmierci była świadoma i przemyślana. Nikt do śmierci mnie nie namawiał. Decyzję o śmierci przez wykrwawienie odpowiadam sam.

### Extract 3

Powiedz – co mam zrobić żebyś chciała być ze mną. Nie chcesz mnie widzieć – tak powiedziałaś – więc nie mogę przyjechać, ale cały czas czekam na taką możliwość *Nigdy* w swoim życiu – nie spodziewałem się takich słów od Ciebie, dlatego jest to taki cios dla mnie, – nie do przeżycia. Wszystkiego mogłem się spodziewać, ale nie tego co mnie spotkało. Cały czas pracowałem byście mieli dobrze. W życiu są różne momenty, ale taki strzał, po tylu latach – coś o czym nawet nie można było pomyśleć.

### Extract 4

Ciężko jest pogodzić się z tym, że kobieta, którą się kocha chce innego mężczyzny i gardzi dawną miłością ani nie ceni podejmowanego dla niej wysiłku – ale wszystko zniosę byle Ci było dobrze. Pozostaję we [city name] by móc pozbierać myśli i spełnić Twoje życzenie ale cały czas czekam na sygnał od Ciebie, bym mógł przyjechać do domu. Rozbiłaś mnie tak, że nie jestem sobą, markuję przed ludźmi, ale nie wiem jak długo dam radę. Boję się przyszłości i tego co może się wydarzyć. Nic nie wiem, ale na wszystko się zgadzam, byle byś była moja i mogła mnie pokochać raz jeszcze.

**Extract 5**

Ciągle jeszcze łudzę się,że wydarzy się coś co mnie zatrzyma. Została jeszcze iskierka nadziei, co prawda ulotna, ale jednak. Ktoś może zapyta dlaczego właśnie tu, w tym miejscu. Powód jest prosty – nie chcę, aby mi ktoś przeszkodził, a tu raczej na pewno tak się nie stanie.

**Extract 6**

Ciągle coś dopisuję bo chcę Was przekonać że życie i zdrowie to jest piękne dopóki się je ma.

**Extract 7**

Jest godzina [exact time] z chwili na chwilę widzę że moje życie nie ma sensu, rozmawiałem przed chwilą z [first_name] i przygnębiła mnie jeszcze bardziej nic nie powiedziała ale chodzi o ton jej głosu był taki nieszczęśliwy, jakby chciała powiedzieć jaka ja jestem nieszczęśliwa z tobą.

**Extract 8**

Dobra. Kochana Siostro koniec użalania się nad sobą i przepraszam że najwięcej zwracam się do Ciebie ale musiałem z kimś porozmawiać.

**Extract 9**

Dzisiaj jest wtorek [date] a ja wykonuję to jutro czyli [date] ponieważ mam jeszcze załatwić jedną sprawę.

**Extract 10**

Udało w końcu zawiesić mi się smycz jeszcze przejdę popojutrze i idę na śmierć.

**Extract 11**

Zabiłaś
Zabiłaś

Zabiłaś
Zabiłaś

**Extract 12**

[first_name] wiesz jak to jest źle jak sobie nie idzie poradzić co ja myślę teraz ja pragnę Cię [first_name] ja wszystko bym Ci wybaczył chciałem się przytulić do Ciebie jak mi tego brakuje

Zdradziłaś mnie dlaczego

Dlaczego mnie zabiłaś

**Extract 13**

I: a jak długo się pani przygotowywała (.) do tego samobójstwa.
R: znaczy ja go odwlekałam jak najbardziej w czasie.

**Extract 14**

no wtedy wtedy się nie chciałem zabić może czasami: nie/ nie/ jakoś m: tak trochę tak trochę chciałem (.) ale z drugiej strony: y: od razu: to: od siebie odrzucam. odrzucałem (.) bo ni: bo w sumie: nie chciałem je: nie chciałbym jej tak zranić.

**Extract 15**

ja tak sobie jedną nogę zamoczyłam i poszłam. [...] i pomyślałam że jeszcze t/ e: jeszcze chwilę poczekam (.) poszłam tam do: (.) m: (.) do: do: dzieci (..) do syna do synowej poszłam do nich i: w międzyczasie jak już piłam kawę przyjechał mój mąż (.) z domu też (.) no on już coś czuwał t/ przeczuwał że ja coś: m/ m/ coś ze mną jest nie tak ale (...) ale y: (.) n/ no nie nie wiedział że ja myślę o czy/ czy/ o czymś takim jak samobójstwo.

**Extract 16**

nie wiem czy tą decyzję podjąłem teraz czy: czy wtedy (..) takie takie bardzo już: jest (to) rozmyte. (..) no bo w każdej chwili mogę jakoś zmienić zdanie. więc w sumie (..) nie wiem czy ten (.) decyzja jest taka podjęta (.) w tym momencie.

**Extract 17**

zacząłem myśleć o tym że: że f: może to dobry pomysł (.) żeby to zrobić (.) wykonać (.) że będzie taki spokój (.) wszystko się skończy (..) no ale to: tak (.) później przestałem o tym myśleć. (.) później się znowu pojawiło (...) a takim: (..) ostatecznym jak gdyby f: f: momentem że mnie (.) pchnęło to do wykonania tego to było ta: y/ informacje że: (..) po prostu ktoś tam coś: miał zrobić obiecał nie zrobił w terminie.

#### Extract 18

weszłam do tej wanny i (.) i: napuściłam wody i t/ i to też tak m: (.) jeszcze stałam i się tak zastanawiałam czy ja dobrze robię (.) myślałam myślałam żeby mężowi powiedzieć może by mnie ws: powstrzymał od tego ale mówię nie. muszę spróbować (.) może się uda teraz. jak nie teraz to już nie wiem.

#### Extract 19

zrobiłam sobie śniadanie też nie mogłam nic jeść (.) i: (..) m: czekałam aż moja mama się obudzi żeby mogła się nim zająć. (..) no i właśnie jak s/ synek poszedł tam do niej do pokoju to: y: poszłam do łazienki zamknęłam się i: wzięłam ten skalpel (..) i też: m/ z (niejasne) stałam. byłam na to nastawiona i: wtedy m/ (.) m/ podcięłam sobie żyły.

#### Extract 20

ja wtenczas spanikowałam [...] se myślę no nie będę czekać do nocy bo jak tata powie bratu to jeszcze mnie tego samego dnia może zawiozą do szpitala. (.) no i wzięłam ten skalpel obustronny.

#### Extract 21

to się nie dzieje tak że człowiek s:taje na moście i po prostu leci sobie (..) [wzdycha] tylko jest ta wewnętrzna walka. przynajmniej u mnie tak było że: (..) u:łamek sekundy decyduje o twoim życiu. (.) że się odepchniesz od mostu lecisz i już jest koniec twojego ży: jest koniec. (.) (bo jak tak powoli to robi:) robi człowiek przygotowuje się i tak dalej to (.) przychodzi zwątpienie. (.) a jeżeli: chce już: tak się zdecydował tak jak ja ostatnio (.) to po prostu (.) (podpiera) idzie idzie idzie i nagle fszu (podpiera) się od mostu i leci. ja c/ ja to tak zrobiłem. w ten sposób. tu była walka: (.) na moście się nie udało.

#### Extract 22

na początku sierpnia: (.) y: z/ (.) zaczęła: się taka: przerwa (.) z moją dziewczyną (.) no i rodzice znowu wyjechali (..) zostawili mnie tam samego w domu (.) i: w sumie się odciąłem tak na tydzień (.) (bo) se siedziałem w domu i nic mi się nie chciało (.) i w ostatni dzień właśnie po prostu: skoczyłem na pętlę (.) na: na drążku się takim (.) do ściany przymocowałem m: tam pasek założyłem po prostu już wisiałem w powietrzu i (.) nie wiem. tak ostatnie takie: (.) wyrzuty sumienia: mnie: popchnęły do tego żeby jednak żyć. i tak palcami się złapałem łó/ łóżka i: (.) zdjąłem tą pętlę i: nie wiem. tam ry/ ryczałem praktycznie do rana.

**Extract 23**

zaczęło się że: nie brałem tabletek e: od jakiegoś czasu (..) no i się powiesiłem. (..) przez tabletki. bo nie brałem.

**Extract 24**

akurat nie wiem czemu to zrobiłem (.) nie wiem. to było jakby p/ to (.) to by/ było trochę jak jakieś przedstawienie (.) że nagrałem s/ samego siebie: y: (połykającego te:) (.) sześćdziesiąt (.) (klonów) (.) klo/ y: ta/ ta/ tabletek Clonazepamu: (.) dwumiligramowych i (.) i: pustą y/ butelkę od pół litra wódki (.) no i s/ wpuściłem to tam: na swojego f/ (.) y/ fejf: facebooka.

**Extract 25**

nie wiem. (.) w sumie czemu to zrobiłem (..) ale czułem się taki s: nie wiem. samotny albo coś choć miałem wszystko w domu (.) y/ chciałem sobie podciąć żyły.

**Extract 26**

ta ostatnia próba [...] jestem może takim seryjnym samobójcą jakimś. może y: (jest) świadczy o tym że trochę (.) i y: jestem i/ nieudacznikiem. co nie (.) albo że: (.) albo że (niejasne) mam jakieś: inne motywy typu (.) y: potrzeba atencji czy: wołanie o pomoc tego typu rzeczy czy: czy nie wiem (.) [...] w sumie nie znam swoich motywów.

# 4 Romanticisation of Suicide

## Introduction

The previous chapter explored agency in acts of suicide. In addition to considering agency in the act of ending one's own life, we also analysed stories of actions that are seemingly marginal to suicide. We also explored agency as a dynamic characteristic of narratives about suicidal experiences, subject to change in the context of telling a story. We argued that stories of waiting for suicide suggested a view of the suicide process that was significantly more complex than previously assumed. Additionally, we argued that the view of suicide in relation to its outcome was too narrow and did not offer sufficient insight into the act.

This chapter continues our examination of constructions of the self in the suicidal situation, where we are interested in stories that romanticise suicide. Specifically, we focus on the narratives in which suicide is constructed as leading to actions or events that are portrayed as desirable or beautiful, while the suicidal individual is positioned as a recipient of those actions or a central figure in the event.

### *Romantic Portrayal of Suicide*

When suicide is portrayed as a heroic or romantic act, it may encourage others to identify with the victim and potentially lead to imitative behaviour. Several researchers agree that sensationalised, glamorous, or detailed reports of suicide can lead to 'copycat' behaviour, where individuals are driven to mimic the publicised suicidal behaviour (Niederkrotenthaler et al., 2012; Stack, 2005).

Copycat suicidal behaviour, a phenomenon known as the Werther effect (Phillips, 1974), describes the increase in suicide rates following media coverage or romanticised portrayals of suicide. The Werther effect has been observed in relation to different types of media, including press and television news, television drama, soap operas, and cinema. However, studies

DOI: 10.4324/9781032672847-4

have shown that the Werther effect is more pronounced when the suicide involves a celebrity. This is because individuals may be more likely to identify with and be influenced by celebrities they admire or feel a connection with (Lueck & Poe, 2023; Ha & Yang, 2021).

Suicides by fictional characters or non-celebrities can also trigger the imitation effect (Domaradzki, 2021). Extensive media coverage and public attention surrounding celebrity suicides can create a sense of connection, potentially leading vulnerable individuals to consider suicide as a viable option (Arendt & Mestas, 2022; Kim et al., 2013). Niederkrotenthaler and co-authors (2020) calculated that reporting the suicidal death of a celebrity appears to increase the number of suicides in the next one to two months by 8–18%. Information about the method of suicide was associated with an 18–44% increase in the risk of suicide by the same method.

Media coverage does not only raise the issue of whose suicides are reported. Researchers have also focused on the characteristics of the stories (agent), individuals' attributes (host), and the social context of the stories (environment) (Gould, 2001). In their book, *Suicide Movies: Social Patterns 1900–2009*, Stack and Bowman (2011) analysed more than 1,377 cinematic suicides in American feature films from 1900 to 2009. They argued that films emphasised external factors influencing suicide, such as rejection of love, financial problems, relationship breakdown, or shame, which are portrayed as root causes of suicide.

Romanticising the reasons behind suicide and presenting them as heroic or rational actions is often accompanied by sensational coverage, glorification, and glamorisation of the deceased. For example, in their study of Indian newspapers, Jain and Kumar (2016) showed that the news was sensationalised in more than 66% of the stories. In over 50% of cases, the news was given front-page coverage, with enlarged headlines or a box to highlight the suicide. Their findings are in line with Domaradzki's review (2021), which highlighted similar observations in many countries. In his observations, a victim was often portrayed as an extraordinary or popular personality, and their suicide was presented as an inevitable or honourable act of bravery. The positive image of suicide was further reinforced by rationalising or romanticising the victim's motives; for example, suicide was described as a result of a terminal or painful illness, financial crisis, job loss, or heartbreak. This can legitimise suicide in the eyes of the public (Domaradzki, 2021).

Parks (2021) suggests significant changes in journalistic practices towards suicide. As he points out, in the early twentieth century, textbooks presented detailed, romantic accounts of suicide, both completed and not, as major news stories. By the turn of the twenty-first century, these reports had been reduced to brief mentions, with the cause of death often avoided in obituaries to respect privacy and prevent copycat attempts. Suicide was no longer treated as a human-interest story (Parks, 2021). Media guidelines are now being encouraged internationally and journalists are becoming more cautious in their reporting practices, avoiding sensationalism, glorification, detailed descriptions of suicide methods, and not presenting suicide as a rational or inexplicable act (McTernan et al., 2018).

Research has shown that a new responsible way of writing about suicide and providing help information alongside non-sensationalised suicide stories is associated with a decrease in copycat suicides following celebrity suicides (Jang et al., 2022; Bohanna & Wang, 2012). Nevertheless, changes in media coverage of suicide are not common (Quarshie et al., 2021), and as Acosta and co-authors (2020) show, working to change suicide coverage requires constant and complex interventions.

Despite significant interest in romanticising suicide in public discourses, we are not aware of any research exploring romanticisation in the 'private' narratives of people engaging in suicidal action. And yet, a romanticised representation of suicide, understood as leading to positive outcomes, is also a characteristic of narratives in suicide notes. By ignoring this aspect of the lived experience of suicide, suicidology misses an important context in which suicide might take place. This chapter attempts to redress this significant research absence.

In this chapter, we focus only on suicide letters. It is the only dataset with stories in which suicide is predicted to lead to positive outcomes. There are three main ways in which suicide is romanticised, and all of them are rendered in instructions left in the suicide letters. First, the person's suicide results in attention from the world. The world must be informed of the suicidal death of the letter author and must observe the event afterwards. Second, those close to the individual taking their life are directed to organise a funeral according to the deceased person's wishes. Finally, authors of suicide letters also direct those close to them to remember them and engage in activities related to such remembrance. We will discuss the romanticisation of the suicide note as an additional dimension of romanticising suicide in the final section of the chapter.

### *Directives*

The notes that we examine in this chapter are mostly in the form of directives, that is to say, their point is to get someone to do something. As Goddard and Wierzbicka (2014) point out, directives are analysed on a spectrum of the force of the instruction. In orders and commands, the strongest of directives, the speaker assumes that the addressee must comply. Requests and advice are weaker in this respect, while in suggestions, the addressee is under no obligation to comply with what the speaker suggests (Wierzbicka, 2003).

For this discussion, we set aside decisions about the exact nature of the directive. We do not wish to decide whether the authors of the notes meant them as orders or instructions. Such a discussion is immaterial from our point of view. What we focus on is the grammatical form of the letters (e.g., clauses in the imperative mood), which does not offer insight into a person's mind.

We are aware, however, that the context of the suicide note, from a person who is about die, makes the request significant. Such directives could be seen as the 'last request' or 'the last wish'. Stereotypically, such 'last requests' are seen outside narratives of suicide (e.g., Heflick, 2005); the fact that a suicide note is the last communication from a person, a request in it, is the last one. We have no evidence, however, whether the letters were so intended or, indeed, so interpreted by their readers. Significantly, some research in suicidology already assumes that the notes are the 'last will' (Jacobs, 1967; Bhatia et al., 2006; Yang & Lester, 2011). Such requests are socially invested with a moral obligation to be complied with. Indeed, as Aries (1981) points out, the moral obligation placed by the 'last will' of someone about to die is common in the 'Western World'.

### The World Will be Looking

In this section, we examine suicide letters in which authors of suicide letters position their death as to be announced and celebrated. Instructions to inform individuals were relatively frequent in the dataset. These were requests to inform close family, such as parents or siblings. In contrast, some letters were requests in which the authors instructed their family to make wider announcements, as in the following notes:

#### Extract 1

Send regards to and inform [a long list of names].

#### Extract 2

You are to inform about my death. [several names] and in general the entire school and all acquaintances in [town name].

#### Extract 3

Bury me in [town name] and inform by obituaries because I want to say goodbye to my acquaintances.

The range of information to be passed increases in the extracts below, from a large group of people, presumably known by the note author, through the entire school and acquaintances in a town, to casting the net wider. Suicide in those notes is far from a private affair; it is something to be broadcast widely. Indeed, the following fragments are requests to inform about the person's death even more widely and the requests are seconded by instructions of how the information is to be conveyed.

**Extract 4**

You are to inform about my death [many names]. For the newspapers and the like give nice fresh pics. New pics are in the computer [file directory name].

**Extract 5**

I would like to thank everyone. I would like, as my last will, for the letter to be read at my funeral. I apologise to my family, friends, but I want them to forgive me for what I did.

The range of announcements in Extract 4 moves from a list of names to newspapers (note the plural) but it is not the range that is the most striking. The request to send 'nice fresh pics' is reminiscent of a PR campaign promoting an individual. Suicidal death becomes an opportunity for the person's 'fifteen minutes of fame'. It becomes an opportunity to launch the note author in the media. Alternatively, and probably more realistically, rendering of the future is conveyed in the note quoted in Extract 5. Suicide is presented as an opportunity to gain a voice, and address everybody in the future.

In the extracts quoted above, suicide is constructed as an event that can and should be announced to the world. Through this, it becomes significant and special, as is the person who took their life. Yet, the specialness of suicide is underscored even more in the following extracts:

**Extract 6**

Please do it for me, my request, I want my entire school to come to my funeral. And [full name].

**Extract 7**

> I would like very much for Mr [last name], a great teacher whom I have always liked, Ms [last name] who is also very important in my life. And [first name] whom I have always treated as a crazy brother.

**Extract 8**

> I would very much like Mr [first name] to make a speech.

In the above extracts, the requests are more restrained (and probably realistic) in their range. Extract 6 is nevertheless a request for a significant number of people to attend the funeral. Extracts 7 and 8 not only request the presence of some people; they give them roles to play. The two extracts request the presence of special guests and thus make the event more special; the central person (the deceased) is honoured in a particular way.

It is worth pointing out the difference between two groups of requests. The requests for communication about the person's death (Extracts 1–4) are made in a very direct, almost impolite way. Note authors use either the imperative mood form translated here as: 'you are to'[1]. Both are on the side of strong directives, which require people to comply. In contrast, the tone of the extracts above (6–8) changes and the requests become more polite. The note authors ask politely rather than command. The two kinds of requests offer interesting insights into the social status or perception of the last request. It seems that the last will cannot simply be commanded and expected to be complied with. Such requests must be made nicely.

In this section, we discussed constructions of suicide as an event leading to a death that is to be announced and viewed. In the first part of the section, we discussed the requests to publicise the person's death, including obituaries in multiple newspapers. In the second part, we briefly showed requests for special people to attend. What is significant in those letters is that suicide is positioned as opening channels of communication widely and to many people.

Suicide has two communicative dimensions. First, it opens a channel of communication for passing information about the person who took their life and their death, which is to be broadcast widely. Second, it also offers the deceased an opportunity to communicate to such audiences. The mirror image of the opportunity to communicate is the opportunity to be noticed and perhaps celebrated. Suicide also offers an opportunity to be the central figure of an event. Both many and special people come to the funeral to acknowledge the death of, by extension, a special person.

One could expect that special people come to specially prepared events. Indeed, authors of suicide notes also have instructions on how to organise the funeral. In the next section, we discuss the requests to make the funeral special.

### *A Special Event*

In this section, we focus on instructions on how to prepare the funeral of the person who took their life. Funerals were romanticised in two ways. On the one hand, note authors requested that the funeral be conducted in a particular way. On the other, they made requests for objects to be buried with them.

We start with extracts in which suicide note authors ask for a particular arrangement of their funeral. Consider the following extracts:

**Extract 9**

> Dad, my only request of you is that let [band name]'s [song title] be played at my funeral in [town name].

**Extract 10**

> Bury me in my uniform with the cap on the casket.

**Extract 11**

> When you read it, don't despair. You will say farewell by my casket. [...] I want to have a beautiful farewell from you all.

From arrangements adorning the event (Extracts 9 and 10), to simply requesting a beautiful service (Extract 11), the note authors' suicides lead to special events. In such requests, the note authors take centre stage in the celebrations that are aimed at celebrating them. However, in the following note, the author goes further in giving detailed instructions about the ornamentation on the tombstone over his grave.

**Extract 12**

> For me definitely the inscription in larger letters: life is beautiful – death a cold kiss. The letters and the cross painted over in silver. Give only the record and my little book. Leave the rest as it is. This will be done by the stonemasons by the cemetery. Give them beforehand so they can hand it out.

Although some of the note speaks to contexts to which we have no access, the note serves the author to design his tombstone. The grandiose inscription painted in silver constructs it as remarkable. Interestingly, the reference to the stonemasonry business suggests that the author had done some preparation, presumably to suggest that their plans were feasible.

If our interpretation as to the function of the reference to the stonemasons is plausible, the reference sets up an interesting contrast with the form of the request. It is an instruction rendered in an imperative mood, suggesting the high force of the directive. It seems, however, that some cajoling is needed.

Several notes requested a burial consisting of scattering the person's ashes. Also here, the beauty of the place is either stressed or implied. Consider:

**Extract 13**

I desire for my ashes to be scattered on Mount [mountain name] ([number] m AMSL).

**Extract 14**

I want to fall on a meadow. Scatter our ashes, I do not want you to pay attention to the place of rest.

**Extract 15**

My last will is for my body to be cremated and the ashes to be scattered in [village name] in the forest. This is the only thing I am asking of you [first name], please make sure of it.

The form of the requests for cremating and scattering of the ashes changes significantly. Instead of directives addressing the recipients of the messages directly, the note authors focus on themselves and their desires. The notes become last wishes and not last requests.

We are unable to explain the change in the linguistic form. We suspect that it is the potential burden that the request places on the addressees, which, in turn, stops the note authors from simply ordering it. This must be seen in the context of Polish funeral practices that are still dominated by burial in the ground. The request therefore goes against the common practice and tradition. This, together with the effort of going, say, to a forest or the top of a mountain, makes the request significant. It is perhaps easier than to express it indirectly through reference to one's wishes.

The last group of fragments we would like to quote here refers to coffin adornments. Consider:

**Extract 16**

Please put our wedding photograph into the coffin, my [football club name] scarf.

**Extract 17**

Put the [football club name] scarf into the coffin. This is my last will.

**Extract 18**

I want to have with me the heart which you gave me.

**Extract 19**

I want to be buried with the teddy bear!! Respect and fulfil my request.

We include these fragments in the chapter on romanticisation as we interpret the requests as having two functions. The first function is set up through the act of asking. As we said at the outset of the chapter, when we ask someone, we put an obligation on them and, at the same time, set up a relationship with them. We believe the notes' additional goal is to construct the note writer as a person who is in relationships with the addressees of the notes. References to a wedding picture, scarf, or teddy bear construct a person who is anchored in the life that the addressees also know. The requests serve as a reminder of the 'little things', the fabric of life, which is about to end. The requested actions to adorn coffins serve, in our view, as tangible reminders of the time spent together. The notes are poignant testimonies of the life that has been, and they put the deceased at the centre of that life.

In this section, we discussed ways in which suicide leads to special things, from arranging the funeral service, through requesting a particular burial, to adorning the coffins. Suicide is a foundation for creating either special events or, as is the case with adornments, special bonds between the diseased and their families. Setting up bonds in the future are focus of the requests in the next section.

## Continuing Bonds

In this section, we discuss a small group of notes in which the request is for those who stay behind to continue their relationship with the note author.

Continuing bonds are usually understood as the presence of an ongoing inner relationship with the deceased person by the bereaved survivor (Shuchter & Zisook, 1993; Field et al., 2003; Schut et al., 2006; Stroebe et al., 2010). The concept of continuing the bond with the deceased was based on the observation of bereaved people made by Klass and co-authors (1996; see also Stroebe, 1992). They observed that the bereaved not only continually seek to gain an understanding of death, but also maintain a connection with the deceased. Thus, they argued, the bond does not have to be broken to 'complete' the process of grieving.

As such, we argue that the continuing bond is not only a psychological state in which an individual finds oneself after the loss of a loved one. We aim to show that such bonds are also requested. Consider:

**Extract 20**

Think of me sometimes, and best once a month bring a white rose to my grave. I will know that you haven't forgotten me.

**Extract 21**

I am asking for one visit a year. Let it be [date], this date is so wonderful for me.

**Extract 22**

I do not want you to visit me every day. Once a year will be enough. I would it to be [date], it is our date.

**Extract 23**

I am sorry for everything. One more thing, bury me in loneliness. I do want crying over my grave. Visit me from time to time.

A paradox is set up in those notes. A person who takes their life, taking themselves out of a relationship, requests for the relationship to continue. Moreover, the relationship is to be marked by special gifts (such as the white rose, as in Extract 20) or acknowledged on special dates. Indirectly, the notes acknowledge that there are socially sanctioned expectations of bereaved families such as social displays of mourning (Taylor, 2009; Neimeyer et al., 2002). Although on the decrease (Bauman, 1998), expectations of what families should and should not do in bereavement continue to exist in today's Poland. Public displays of mourning such as black clothing and ribbons are still common, as are expectations of visiting and tending the deceased relative's grave. In such letters, once again, suicide is not an end. It is the beginning of a new relationship with those left behind. Let us now consider one last example:

**Extract 24**

My clothes, notebooks, book, I want you to take it all. Our teddy bears, our photographs, notes (they are in the blue box under the desk, the one on the top). Get the photographs from [place name] developed, cover yourself with my little blanket. Think about me. But not too much. Live!

There is an apparent ambivalence in the note. The author suggests a significant presence in the life of the note addressee. The request for presence is conveyed in strong imperatives. The initial focus on the author's will is replaced with clauses with verbs in the imperative mood. Yet, right at the end of the note, the author undermines the strength of the directive. The note constructs a beautiful life for the addressee, covered by the blanket, looking at the picture, and thinking about the deceased author of the note. In this context, the weakening of the message towards the end, we suggest, is only apparent. Rather, we see it as an expression of care.

## Farewell

So far, we have discussed how suicide is romanticised in suicide notes through directives wishing for something positive or desirable to result from suicide. We discussed suicide as a means of opening communication channels, and we showed romanticisation through wishing and designing a special event commemorating the person who took their life. Finally, we discussed constructions of relationships enduring beyond suicide. In all of them, the assumption was that the suicide either had already happened or would have happened and the events planned happened after the suicidal act.

In this section, we suggest a different kind of romanticisation. The notes also make both the note and the time of writing extraordinary. We end our discussion in this chapter with a brief account of suicide notes that are presented as special messages. Note authors stress that what was happening to them was significant, emotional, and grand.

Consider these two groups of notes. First we discuss those that refer to the notes themselves:

**Extract 25**

This letter is a farewell and at the same time my last will.

**Extract 26**

My final farewell with my family.

**Extract 27**

My beloved husband, and beloved parents, we are saying goodbye forever.

The drama of the final farewell is underscored by the emotionality of writing. Now, consider:

**Extract 28**

What I have written here has been sprinkled with the tears of my despair.

**Extract 29**

I do not know what more I should write you [plural], because it is hard to leave people one loves. And my heart is breaking now.

We suggest that the notes are intended to stress the significance of the moment because one can commonsensically assume that such messages can be considered superfluous. Suicide notes are the last messages and are likely to be written with emotions running relatively high. The addressees can hardly make a mistake interpreting the notes left by the deceased family member. The time of writing will likely be assumed as dramatic, as a suicide note is an extraordinary message to receive. After all, it is likely to contain the last words of a person who has just taken their life. This seems significant enough.

This is why we looked for another explanation of such messages. The idea that such messages serve to romanticise the act seems plausible. Furthermore, reference to the drama might also be a way of suggesting that the decision to take one's life was not taken lightly. The note is used to convey the writer's anguish, while the writer constructs themselves as caught in an extraordinary situation.

Consider another group of extracts in which the stakes are even higher. References to bad handwriting serve as an introduction to the author's emotional state:

**Extract 30**

I am sorry for misspellings and the handwriting but I cannot calm down writing this letter. My hands are shaking because of the worries. Why did it all have to end like that.

**Extract 31**

I am sorry for my handwriting, but I am shaking all over. I cannot, I wanted to fix it all, please.

**Extract 32**

I might be writing illegibly, because my hands are shaking, but it does not matter.

Apologies for the handwriting in a suicide note seem astonishing. Surely, one does not need to apologise for not taking care to write neatly when writing their last words. Thus, we think that references to handwriting are a way of both introducing the writers' emotionality and, at the same time, offering evidence for it. In a nutshell, such notes underscore the significance of the time.

These typical extracts contain two parts. Intuitively, one is the apology for the handwriting; the other is the explanation, or perhaps, justification of the handwriting. The justification constructs the time of writing as momentous, significant, and full of emotions. This is not ordinary writing; this is writing that simply cannot be neat and beautiful, even if the authors wanted it so. An additional point in Extract 32 is worth making here. As the man explains writing illegibly, his hands are shaking, but he adds, 'But it does not matter.' The letter must be written, and no difficulty will stop the man.

We would like to end this section with one last extract:

**Extract 33**

I [first name] am killing myself.

The note is extraordinary. It is reminiscent of performative sentences first described by Austin (1962), who proposed that some utterances do not so much tell us about something, but, instead, do something. And so, if you say, given the right circumstances, 'I (hereby) take you to be my wife/husband', 'I sentence you to death', you also do this. In other words, you get married or you sentence the person to die. Later it also became clear that sentences such as, 'I promise you', 'I forgive you', or 'I apologise' are a promise, an act of forgiving, and an apology, respectively (Searle, 1969).

Writing 'I kill myself' will not actually kill you, so there must be another reason for writing it. As we argued elsewhere (Galasiński, 2017), we propose that the note is the beginning of suicide; it invokes the suicide and (thereby) initiates it. The note above is constitutive of the act of suicide, making it more significant and extraordinary. Our argument positions the note as a dramatic part of the suicidal act that follows it. The letter's main function, we suggest, is to underscore the moment of suicide, to stress the drama of the situation.

This section briefly discussed suicide notes as a means to romanticise the time before the suicidal act. We argue that introducing elements that can be assumed to be true into the notes serves primarily to portray the act and the preceding time as extraordinary.

## Conclusion

In this chapter, we discussed ways in which suicide is romanticised in suicide notes. There are three main ways in which this is done. First, people writing suicide notes request for their death to be publicised widely—others should learn about the person and celebrate the deceased after their death. Second, note authors ask for their funerals to be arranged in a particular way. Third, these requests are often accompanied by instructions on how the attendees must celebrate. All three ways of romanticisation are done through directives. The note authors offer instructions to their close ones on how they should proceed after their death.

The first question we asked of the results is their source. We were particularly interested in the instructions for informing the media about the person's death. Below is an excerpt from a note:

### Extract 34

> You are to inform about my death [many names]. For the newspapers and the like give nice fresh pics. New pics are in the computer [file directory name].

This extract, which we quoted earlier, looks more like a sketch for a PR campaign and not a suicide note.

Of course, we have no access to the person's thoughts and wishes behind the note. Yet, it is difficult not to see some affinities with the romanticised media coverage of some suicides. The issue for us, however, is the nature of the relationship between media coverage and the wish to advertise one's death.

Suicidology is mostly interested in the risk groups after celebrity suicide and the results are mixed apart from general statements that those who are vulnerable or at risk may be more likely to engage in copycat suicidal behaviour if they are exposed to narratives that idealise or romanticise suicide. It has been shown that younger adults with depression are particularly vulnerable to the influence of celebrity suicides (Fink et al., 2018; Guinovart et al., 2023).

However, in their study of the Werther effect following the suicides of three Korean celebrity singers, Kim and co-authors (2023) found that women had higher rates of copycat suicide. Conversely, Fink and co-authors (2018) showed that after the death of Robin Williams, the rate of copycat suicide was higher among men. Perhaps, as suggested by Fu and Chan (2013), the rate of copycat suicides may vary depending on the coverage of and circumstances at the time of the celebrity suicide. The Werther effect mostly applies to two types of celebrities: entertainers (i.e., music and film stars) and political figures (Domaradzki, 2021).

We would like to suggest a different possibility. The link with celebrities might not always be identification with the celebrity; instead, it could be the wish to have one's suicidal death made public. In other words, suicide and its publicisation are a means to claim the centre stage and become the focus of attention, however brief.

Our argument is supported by internet debates on how to write a suicide note. Phrased as 'how to write a good suicide note', such discussions are concerned with the impact suicide notes might have. Regardless of whether discussants are suicidal or not, they position suicide notes not as simple goodbyes, but as statements. Indeed, some answers to questions of this kind suggest writing small treatises on the world and its ills. In such a way, we suggest that at least some copycat suicides are not so much imitating a previous suicide, but they are seeking a similar kind of public impact. Unfortunately, research cannot offer any other empirical evidence apart from text-based.

Our arguments lead to several issues for suicide prevention and what it focuses on. One wonders, for example, about the extent a campaign making the wishes of publicity realistic could be preventative of some suicides. It is highly unlikely that a non-celebrity's suicide would be given coverage similar to that of a famous person, thus making it clear might have some protective impact. Such arguments suggest the importance of research into romanticisation. As noted earlier, we have not found any previous research into the romanticisation of suicide in 'private' narratives. The results we report here suggest that romanticisation strategies offer important insight into the relevancies and functions of suicide.

For example, our data suggest that romantic representation of suicide consistently reaches out into the future. Tragically, all those futures in the suicide notes are unlikely to happen. Driving the message that suicide is an end, rather than a beginning, might well be a strategy worth pursuing in prevention.

Both romanticisation of suicide and discussions on how to write a suicide note also point to the complexity of suicide notes themselves. Often assumed to give insight into the suicidal mind (see a full discussion in Galasiński, 2017), suicide notes can be seen as having several communicative and social functions. They are not simple farewells. Instead, they are strategic pieces of communication that give their authors opportunities to realise their goals. The final question we would like to raise here is whether romantic representations of suicide could be seen as attempting to make it more acceptable. Is a beautiful funeral or media coverage aimed at making suicide less tragic?

At the moment, we have no answer to such a question but, as we discussed in the previous chapter, suicide's acceptability has increased. While we think that romanticisation in narratives of lived experience is unlikely to contribute to its macro-level acceptability, we think a relationship between growing acceptability and romanticisation is worth exploring further. Romantic representation might well be a result of the growing acceptability, while in the local context, romanticisation might be aimed at making a particular suicide less dramatic. This, again, raises important issues for prevention strategies.

In the next chapter, we start exploring narratives of relationships in which suicidal individuals find themselves. We want to put a question mark on the assumption that suicide is located in the individual, their vulnerabilities, decision-making processes, and personality traits. Individuals focus on others in their narratives about suicide. This is evident both in suicide notes, where the narrative precedes the suicidal act, and in the post-attempt interviews, where the narrative comes after the attempt. We contrast the two datasets to determine whether there are differences in how the self is constructed depending on its position within the suicide timeline.

## Note

1 This is how we render the Polish phrase '*mieć* + infinitive', which is a very strong directive implying both the power to make it and some power over the addressee. Our linguistic competences suggest that the phrase is more direct and less polite than the instruction given through the form of the imperative mood.

## References

Acosta, F. J., Rodríguez, C. J., Cejas, M. R., Ramallo-Fariña, Y., & Fernandez-Garcimartin, H. (2020). Suicide coverage in the digital press media: Adherence to World Health Organization guidelines and effectiveness of different

interventions aimed at media professionals. *Health Communication*, *35*(13), 1623–1632. https://doi.org/10.1080/10410236.2019.1654176
Arendt, F., & Mestas, M. (2022). Celebrity suicide of a pre-World War I spy. *Crisis, 43*(2), 112–118. https://doi.org/10.1027/0227-5910/a000762
Aries, P. (1981). *The hour of our death*. Alfred A. Knopf.
Austin, J. L. (1962). *How to do things with words*. Clarendon Press.
Bauman, Z. (1998). Postmodern adventures of life and death. In G. Scambler & P. Higgs (Eds.), *Modernity, medicine and health* (pp. 217–232). Routledge.
Bhatia, M. S., Verma, S. K., & Murty, O. P. (2006). Suicide notes: Psychological and clinical profile. *The International Journal of Psychiatry in Medicine*, *36*(2), 163–170. https://doi.org/10.2190/5690-CMGX-6A1C-Q28H
Bohanna, I., & Wang, X. (2012). Media guidelines for the responsible reporting of suicide: A review of effectiveness. *Crisis*, *33*(4), 190–198. https://doi.org/10.1027/0227-5910/a000137
Domaradzki, J. (2021). The Werther effect, the Papageno effect or no effect? A literature review. *International Journal of Environmental Research and Public Health*, *18*(5), 2396. https://doi.org/10.3390/ijerph18052396
Field, N. P., Gal-Oz, E., & Bonanno, G. A. (2003). Continuing bonds and adjustment at 5 years after the death of a spouse. *Journal of Consulting and Clinical Psychology, 71*(1), 110–117. https://doi.org/10.1037/0022-006X.71.1.110
Fink, D. S., Santaella-Tenorio, J., & Keyes, K. M. (2018). Increase in suicides the months after the death of Robin Williams in the US. *PloS One*, *13*(2), e0191405. https://doi.org/10.1371/journal.pone.0191405
Fu, K. W., & Chan, C. H. (2013). A study of the impact of thirteen celebrity suicides on subsequent suicide rates in South Korea from 2005 to 2009. *PloS One*, *8*(1), e53870. https://doi.org/10.1371/journal.pone.0053870
Galasiński, D. (2017). *Discourses of men's suicide notes: A qualitative analysis*. Bloomsbury Publishing.
Goddard, C., & Wierzbicka, A. (2014). *Words and meanings: Lexical semantics across domains, languages, and cultures*. Oxford University Press.
Gould, M. S. (2001). Suicide and the media. *Annals of the New York Academy of Sciences*, *932*, 200–224. https://doi.org/10.1111/j.1749-6632.2001.tb05807.x
Guinovart, M., Cobo, J., González-Rodríguez, A., Parra-Uribe, I., & Palao, D. (2023). Towards the influence of media on suicidality: A systematic review of Netflix's 'Thirteen Reasons Why'. *International Journal of Environmental Research and Public Health*, *20*(7), 5270. https://doi.org/10.3390/ijerph20075270
Ha, J., & Yang, H. S. (2021). The Werther effect of celebrity suicides: Evidence from South Korea. *PLoS ONE*, *16*(4), e0249896. https://doi.org/10.1371/journal.pone.0249896
Heflick, N. A. (2005). Sentenced to die: Last statements and dying on death row. *OMEGA-Journal of Death and Dying*, *51*(4), 323–336.
Jacobs, J. (1967). A phenomenological study of suicide notes. *Social Problems*, *15*(1), 60–72.
Jain, N., & Kumar, S. (2016). Is suicide reporting in Indian newspapers responsible? A study from Rajasthan. *Asian Journal of Plpsychiatry*, *24*, 135–138. https://doi.org/10.1016/j.ajp.2016.09.012

Jang, J., Myung, W., Kim, S., Han, M., Yook, V., Kim, E. J., & Jeon, H. J. (2022). Effect of suicide prevention law and media guidelines on copycat suicide of general population following celebrity suicides in South Korea, 2005–2017. *The Australian and New Zealand Journal of Psychiatry*, *56*(5), 542–550. https://doi.org/10.1177/00048674211025701

Kim, J. H., Nam, C. M., Park, S., Cho, J., Kim, S. J., Choi, J. W., & Cho, E. (2013). The Werther effect of two celebrity suicides: An entertainer and a politician. *PLoS One*, *8*(12), e84876. https://doi.org/10.1371/journal.pone.0084876

Kim, L. H., Lee, G. M., Lee, W. R., & Yoo, K. B. (2023). The Werther effect following the suicides of three Korean celebrities (2017–2018): An ecological time-series study. *BMC Public Health*, *23*(1), 1173. https://doi.org/10.1186/s12889-023-16080-1

Klass, D., Silverman, P. R., & Nickman, S. L. (Eds.). (1996). *Continuing bonds: New understandings of grief*. Taylor & Francis.

Lueck, J. A., & Poe, M. (2023). Werther or Papageno? Examining the effects of news reports of celebrity suicide versus non-celebrity peer suicide on intentions to seek help among vulnerable young adults. *Suicide and Life-Threatening Behavior*, *53*(6), 1038–1054. https://doi.org/10.1111/sltb.13004

McTernan, N., Spillane, A., Cully, G., Cusack, E., O'Reilly, T., & Arensman, E. (2018). Media reporting of suicide and adherence to media guidelines. *International Journal of Social Psychiatry*, *64*(6), 536–544. https://doi.org/10.1177/0020764018784

Neimeyer, R. A., Prigerson, H. G., & Davies, B. (2002). Mourning and meaning. *American Behavioral Scientist*, *46*(2), 235–251. https://doi.org/10.1177/000276402236676

Niederkrotenthaler, T., Braun, M., Pirkis, J., Till, B., Stack, S., Sinyor, M., Tran, U. S., Voracek, M., Cheng, Q., Arendt, F., Scherr, S., Yip, P. S. F., & Spittal, M. J. (2020). Association between suicide reporting in the media and suicide: Systematic review and meta-analysis. *BMJ (Clinical research ed.)*, *368*, m575. https://doi.org/10.1136/bmj.m575

Niederkrotenthaler, T., Fu, K. W., Yip, P. S., Fong, D. Y., Stack, S., Cheng, Q., & Pirkis, J. (2012). Changes in suicide rates following media reports on celebrity suicide: A meta-analysis. *Journal of Epidemiology and Community Health*, *66*(11), 1037–1042. https://doi.org/10.1136/jech-2011-200707

Parks, P. (2021). From sensation to stigma: Changing standards for suicide coverage in US journalism textbooks, 1894–2016. *Journalism*, *22*(6), 1375–1392. https://doi.org/10.1177/146488491984192

Phillips, D. P. (1974). The influence of suggestion on suicide: Substantive and theoretical implications of the Werther effect. *American Sociological Review*, *39*(3), 340–354. https://doi.org/10.2307/2094294

Quarshie, E. N., Andoh-Arthur, J., Asante, K. O., & Asare-Doku, W. (2021). Online media reporting of suicidal behaviour in Ghana: Analysis of adherence to the WHO guidelines. *The International Journal of Social Psychiatry*, *67*(3), 251–259. https://doi.org/10.1177/0020764020919787

Schut, H. A. W., Stroebe, M. S., Boelen, P. A., & Zijerveld, A. M. (2006). Continuing relationships with the deceased: Disentangling bonds and grief. *Death Studies*, *30*(8), 757–766. https://doi.org/10.1080/07481180600850666

Searle, J. R. (1969). *Speech acts: An essay in the philosophy of language* (Vol. 626). Cambridge University Press.
Shuchter, S. R., & Zisook, S. (1993). The course of normal grief. In M. S. Stroebe, W. Stroebe, & R. O. Hansson (Eds.), *Handbook of bereavement: Theory, research, and intervention* (pp. 23–43). Cambridge University Press. https://doi.org/10.1017/CBO9780511664076.003
Stack, S. (2005). Suicide in the media: A quantitative review of studies based on non-fictional stories. *Suicide & Life-Threatening Behavior*, *35*(2), 121–133. https://doi.org/10.1521/suli.35.2.121.62877
Stack, S., & Bowman, B. (2011). *Suicide movies: Social patterns 1900–2009*. Hogrefe Publishing GmbH.
Stroebe, M. (1992). Coping with bereavement: A review of the grief work hypothesis. *Omega*, 26, 19–42.
Stroebe, M., Schut, H., & Boerner, K. (2010). Continuing bonds in adaptation to bereavement: Toward theoretical integration. *Clinical Psychology Review*, *30*(2), 259–268. https://doi.org/10.1016/j.cpr.2009.11.007
Taylor, L. (2009). *Mourning dress*. Routledge.
Wierzbicka, A. (2003). *Cross-cultural pragmatics: The semantics of human interaction*. Walter de Gruyter.
Yang, B., & Lester, D. (2011). The presentation of the self: A hypothesis about suicide notes. *Suicidology Online*, *2*, 75–79.

## Appendix

### Extract 1

Send regards to and inform [a long list of names].

### Extract 2

Macie poinformować o mojej śmierci:

[names] I ogólnie całą szkołę i wszystkich znajomych z [town name]

### Extract 3

Pochowajcie mnie w [town name] i powiadomcie klepsydrami bo chcę się pożegnać ze znajomymi.

### Extract 4

Macie poinformować o mojej śmierci: [many names]. Do gazet itp. dawajcie świeże ładne foty, nowe foty są w kompie [file directory name]

**Extract 5**

Chciałbym podziękować każdemu. Prosiłbym jako ostatnią wolę aby ten list był odczytany na moim pogrzebie przepraszam swoją rodzinę kolegów przyjaciół ale chcę aby mi wybaczyli to co zrobiłem

**Extract 6**

Zróbcie dla mnie prośbę chcę żeby na mój pogrzeb przyszła cała moja szkoła i [first_name] [last_name].

**Extract 7**

Bardzo bym chciał aby na pogrzebie byli pan [lps_acr_first_name] [last_name] znakomity nauczyciel którego zawsze obdarzałem wielką sympatią, Pani [lps_acr_first_name] [last_name] też bardzo ważną osobą w moim życiu no i [first_name] którego zawsze traktowałem jako swego szalonego brata.

**Extract 8**

Bardzo bym chciał aby pan [first_name] wygłosił przemówienie

**Extract 9**

Tato moja jedyna prośba do Ciebie niech na moim pogrzebie w [town name] zagrają piosenkę [ song name] – [band name]

**Extract 10**

Pochowajcie mnie w mundurze z moją czapką na trumnie

**Extract 11**

Kiedy to przeczytasz nie załamuj się po prostu pożegnasz mnie przy mojej trumnie. [...] I chcę mieć piękne pożegnanie od Was wszystkich.

**Extract 12**

Dla mnie w powiększeniu koniecznie napis. ŻYCIE JEST PIĘKNE – ŚMIERĆ ZIMNYM POCAŁUNKIEM. Litery i krzyż pomalowane srebrzanką. Dać tylko płytę i moją książeczkę – resztę zostawić jak było. To wykona zakład kamieniarski pod cmentarzem firma. Zgłosić przed pogrzebem aby to rozdali.

**Extract 13**

PRAGNĘ ABY MOJE PROCHY BYŁY ROZSYPANE NA [mountain name] [number] m n.p.m.

**Extract 14**

Chcę spaść na łąkę. Rozrzuć nasze prochy, nie chcę, żebyś przywiązywał się do miejsca (spoczynku)

**Extract 15**

moim ostatnim życzeniem jest aby moje ciało spalić a prochy rozsypać na Soputku w lesie o to jedno Cię [first_name] proszę dopilnuj tego

**Extract 16**

Proszę do mojej trumny włóż nasze zdjęcie ślubne, mój szalik [football club name]

**Extract 17**

Do mojej trumny dajcie szalik [football club name] To jest moja ostatnia wola!!!

**Extract 18**

Chcę przy sobie mieć serduszko które mi kiedyś podarowałeś.

**Extract 19**

Chcę być pochowana z misiem!!
Uszanujcie i spełnijcie moją prośbę!

**Extract 20**

Wspominaj mnie czasami, a najlepiej raz w miesiącu przynieś na mój grób białą różę będę wiedział że o mnie nie zapomniałaś.

**Extract 21**

proszę jedynie o wizytę raz w roku i niech to będzie [date],
ta data jest dla mnie cudowna.

**Extract 22**

Nie chcę żebyś odwiedzał mnie co dzień... wystarczy mi jeden raz w roku i chciałabym żeby to był [date] nasza data...

**Extract 23**

Przepraszam za wszystko i jeszcze jedno pochowaj mnie w samotności
nie chcę płaczu nad moim grobem. Odwiedź mnie
od czasu do czasu

**Extract 24**

Moje ubrania, zeszyty, książki – chcę żebyś zabrał wszystko. Nasze misie, nasze zdjęcia, zapiski (są w niebieskim pudełku pod biurkiem, tym na górze). Wywołaj zdjęcia z Bieszczad, okrywaj się moim kocykiem. Myśl o mnie. Ale nie za dużo – żyj.

**Extract 25**

Ten list jest pożegnaniem i jednocześnie testamentem.

**Extract 26**

Moje Ostateczne Pożegnanie z Rodziną

**Extract 27**

Kochany mój mężu i kochani rodzice żegnamy się już na wieki.

**Extract 28**

To co tu napisałem zostało skropione łzami mej rozpaczy.

**Extract 29**

Nie wiem co mam Wam więcej napisać bo trudno jest zostawić ludzi których się kocha i serce mi w tym momencie pęka

**Extract 30**

Przepraszam za błędy i pismo lecz nie mogę się opanować pisząc ten list. Ręce mi drżą ze zgryzoty. Dlaczego tak to źle się musiało skończyć (to wszystko).

**Extract 31**

Przepraszam za pismo ale już się cały trzepię nie mogę chciałem wszystko naprawić proszę

**Extract 32**

Mogę pisać trochę nieczytelnie, bo mi się cholernie ręce trzęsą, no ale nieważne.

**Extract 33**

Ja [first_name] się zabijam

**Extract 34**

Macie poinformować o mojej śmierci: [many names]. Do gazet itp. dawajcie świeże ładne foty, nowe foty są w kompie [file directory name]

# 5 Self in Interaction

## Introduction

In the previous chapter, we discussed romanticisation of suicide. In contrast to the suicidological research tradition, which focuses solely on romanticisation of suicide in public discourses, we examined the romantic representation of suicide in farewell letters. We examined strategies of 'private' romanticisation of suicide and argued that understanding representations of suicide as positive and leading to desirable outcomes was an important aspect of suicide prevention. This chapter is the first in which we explore narrated relationships in which the suicidal individual finds themselves. We examine here how those who engaged in suicidal action construct themselves in their stories about suicide. It is common in theories and research on suicide to place the individual at the centre of the act, focusing on personal and psychological factors leading to suicide. They highlight the role of individual vulnerabilities, decision-making processes, and personality traits in shaping suicidal behaviour.

Our research puts a question mark on such assumptions. Individuals focus on others in their stories about suicide, both in the suicide notes, where the narrative comes before the suicidal act, and in the post-attempt interviews, where the narrative comes after the attempt. In this chapter, we contrast the two datasets to examine whether there are differences in how the self is constructed depending on its position on the suicide timeline.

The argument we make in this chapter is two-fold. First, we propose that when referring to suicide, people attempting to, or taking their lives, consistently position themselves and the action in a relationship with their close ones. The second argument is that suicide offers a negative identity, that is, an identity of what one is not or does not want to be. Suicide introduces a dilemma into the stories of those either committing or attempting to commit suicide. As such, suicide is both espoused and rejected.

We end the chapter with a discussion of the most common dimension of suicide behaviour—thwarted belongingness—which constructs suicide

DOI: 10.4324/9781032672847-5

as resulting from losing a connection. However, the data we examined showed that suicide is consistently represented in relationship-affirming narratives. In other words, suicide stories are ones in which connectedness is emphasised and acknowledged.

## Relationships and Thwarted Identity

Suicide and suicide attempts almost always take place within a family. Close ones have a significant impact on an individual's overall risk of suicide and, conversely, suicide of a loved one has a significant impact on those close to them. Those who live on their own are at heightened risk of suicide attempts, compared to those living with family members (Denney, 2010). Yet when suicide happens, it is estimated that between six family members and up to 135 individuals may be affected (Cerel et al., 2019).

Frey and Cerel's (2015) narrative review of family factors in suicide risk showed that much of the research focused on family structure. Living alone may result in heightened feelings of loneliness, lack of social support, and depression, all of which are associated with an increased risk of suicide (Niu et al., 2020). Narita and co-authors (2024) argue that living alone can result in social isolation and loneliness, conditions that are strongly correlated with a sense of thwarted belongingness, which further exacerbates suicide risk.

The type and quality of the relationship in the family are also important. Marriage, cohabitation or having close relationships with family members have been consistently associated with a lower risk of suicide, while being divorced, separated, widowed, or single is associated with an increased risk of suicide, while (Shaw et al., 2021; Purcell et al., 2012; Narita et al., 2024; Wyder et al., 2009; Yip et al., 2015). Parenthood has also been associated with reduced suicide risk (Shaw et al., 2021), but Cerel (as cited in Zareian & Klonsky, 2020) found that conflict with children, or with a spouse regarding the children, often preceded parents' suicidal behaviour.

According to Frey and Cerel (2015), conflict is one of the most extensively explored areas when examining the relationship between family and suicide. Conflicts with parents, friends, and romantic partners increase suicide risk among adolescents (Frey & Cerel, 2015; see also: Eslava et al., 2023). Similarly, for adults, conflicts with romantic partners have been consistently identified as a significant risk factor for suicide (Kazan et al., 2016). A recent study by Carter and co-authors (2024) found that on the day of a suicide attempt, 27.3% of individuals reported issues with their romantic partners. The authors underline the immediate impact of relationship problems on suicidal behaviours and argue that conflicts with romantic partners can act as a unique predictor of suicide attempts on the same day (Carter et al., 2024).

The results of the research described above are reflected in the theoretical concepts. These range from Durkheim's egoistic suicide as a result of a lack of social integration or belonging, leading to feelings of isolation and alienation, which may contribute to an increased risk of suicide, to contemporary models of suicide rooted in the ideation-to-action framework, for example, the Interpersonal Theory of Suicide (IPTS) or the Three-Step Theory (3ST).

Of particular relevance here is the concept of thwarted belongingness, which the Interpersonal Theory of Suicide identifies as critical to understanding suicidal ideation and behaviour (Joiner, 2005; van Orden et al., 2005; van Orden et al., 2010). Thwarted belongingness is the experience of feeling alienated, isolated, and unsupported by friends, family, or other valued social circles. It refers to a loss of sense of belonging or lack of social connectedness that may increase vulnerability to suicidal thoughts and actions. Thwarted belongingness is often associated with other psychological states, such as perceived burdensomeness; together, these factors may lead to the emergence of suicidal ideation (Brochu et al., 2021).

A similar meaning is attached to the concept of connectedness in the Three Step Theory (Klonsky & May, 2015). Connectedness, especially social connectedness, plays a protective role against suicidal ideation and behaviour. According to the Three-Step Theory, suicidal ideation is the result of a combination of pain and hopelessness. What happens with suicidal ideation depends on the relationship between pain and connectedness. If connectedness predominates, for example, related to people, roles, or other values in life, then the person will continue to live despite the pain. However, if the pain predominates, or is so strong that it excludes connectedness, then suicidal ideation becomes stronger. In such a state, if the individual can act on suicidal ideation, they can move from thought to action.

However, this chapter aims to show a more nuanced view of suicide and relationships. Not only are relationships part of the suicide process but consistently, those engaged in suicidal behaviour consistently construct themselves as in relationships, which, sometimes, are represented as surviving suicide.

We also analyse both data sets. However, we only focus on how the self is represented in narratives about the suicide itself. So, we only looked for fragments where the note writer or interviewee talked about suicide and taking their own life. As such, we exclude all stories that talk about unhappiness, relationships, poor health, and other circumstances.

In such a way, we constructed a subset of the data with fragments in which taking one's life was mentioned. This was done explicitly, for example, through references to the process of taking one's life, or of dying, or to death. However, we also included implicit references to suicide. We included such verbs as 'departing' or 'leaving' as contextual references to dying or asking for forgiveness for 'what happened' as referring to suicide.

Similarly, references to 'the act' in the suicide notes were the most frequent reference to suicide.

Our discussion goes as follows: first, we discuss references to dying or killing oneself in the suicide notes. We argue that such references consistently construct a relationship that is affirmed by the notes. We also discuss narratives of people who made a serious attempt on their lives. Such narratives, we argue, are full of ambivalence about the suicide itself, but they also refer to existing relationships.

### Unending Interactions

When authors of suicide notes directly refer to their suicide, the notes consistently construct an existing relationship with those who are left behind. The notes construct unending relationships and interactions that last through suicide. Consider first the following three extracts that render well the dominant group representations.

#### Extract 1

I love you very much and I apologise for what I have done. But the situation got the better of me and I cannot cope with it. Forgive me all and especially you my beloved [first name].

#### Extract 2

I am sorry for everything, but I cannot live like that. My kidneys hurt.
I am really sorry.
I love you [addressing many] and I am sorry.
I love you, my wife.

#### Extract 3

I love you, I love you, I love you. I am sorry for what I have done. It has caused you pain and despair, but after a time you will reach the conclusion that it was best this way. I have always said that I do not want to hurt anyone and this is why I have done what I have done.

There are two main ways in which relationships are reaffirmed in suicide letters: apologies and confessions of love, often done in the same narrative, such as in the extracts above. Even though love refers to an emotional commitment towards a person and an apology implies responsibility for something negative, both acts of communication construct a relationship of value and importance. Loving someone makes them a 'significant other';

an apology implies the wish to obtain forgiveness. One does not want or need forgiveness from someone they do not care about.

Both acts of communication serve as narrative-creating devices. In Extract 1, a confession and an apology form superordinate clauses[1] that introduce the euphemistic references to suicide. A similar construction can be seen in Extract 3. After the initial four clauses expressing love, it is the apology that introduces the implicit reference to suicide. Extract 2, on the other hand, is different; the reference to suicide ('everything') is not in a clause and is disambiguated through the following coordinate clause.

These grammatical forms are significant as they represent the relationship between the note author and their addressees as the dominant perspective in the accounts. In such notes, suicide is depicted through the eyes of those who experience it. Love and contrition stand on their own in the account, while suicide is secondary. Below, is another group of extracts showing a similar pattern, although this time the letter authors refer to forgiveness.

**Extract 4**

I do not know if you and the children will forgive me for this. But I am asking, please, forgive [addressing many]; forgive me what I have done to you. Farewell [addressing many].

**Extract 5**

I apologise to all for what I have done. [First name], forgive me, please. I love you very much. No one is to blame for what has happened.

**Extract 6**

Forgive me for what I have done and all the hurt I have caused you. Call my doctor [last name] and say that I apologise that I failed her. I wish you happiness without me. I also apologise to my daughter [first name] for what I have done and all the hurt from me. I apologise to those I have failed, all of you.

Extract 4 introduces suicide through a reference to forgiveness; Extract 5 starts with an apology that is followed by a plea for forgiveness. Extract 6 also begins with a clause in the imperative mood asking for forgiveness.

We would like to make two additional points about the apologies quoted in the extracts. First, these are not ordinary apologies. They are grammatically highlighted to introduce the suicidal act and are constructed as full of importance and significance. They are also accompanied by confessions of ('great', 'greatest', 'undying') love and they contain requests for forgiveness. Even though they suggest that something of much significance is either about to happen or already happened, they are used to construct the primacy of the relationship represented in the note. In other words, it is not the suicide that seems key in the notes; it is the relationship that is made to last in the texts.

Second, an apology is a communicative act that requires a response from the addressee, ideally, forgiveness or some other act of absolution. The apologising authors of the notes position themselves at the mercy of those who must accept this 'special apology' and grant them forgiveness. However, those who apologise in a suicide note will never know what the upshot of their communicative action would be. Moreover, the addressees will never get the opportunity to respond. As the apology will never be completed, the relationship between the one who apologises and the recipient of the apology will continue. The response will always be due to happen, and the addressee of the apology will always owe a response.

This argument ties in well with one made earlier that suicide is often rendered as non-final (Galasiński, 2017). For example, farewell letters are laden with confessions of love that will continue well into the future after the death of the person who took their life. For example:

**Extract 7**

I will always love you.

**Extract 8**

I love you. You will always be in my heart.

**Extract 9**

I will love [her] till the end of her life.

In these letters, the authors promise eternal love as if suicide would not put an end to the person's feelings. Significantly, the fragments do not refer to some abstract love; they are about one person's love to another that will continue to exist, surviving the former's death. We understand that such assurances or promises of love are anchored in the narrative of romantic love that never ends. However, the never-ending love is constructed well beyond the loving person's physical existence. The exception is Extract 9, which seems to make the everlasting more concrete and places the time limit on the loved person's death. What is important for the discussion here is that the confessions seem to be maintaining a relationship with the person left behind.

In some cases, constructions of the enduring relationship go beyond confessions of love. For example, the author of the note below offers considerably more:

**Extract 10**

> My love, I love you very much, but I have no more strength. I will always be with you in spirit. Forgive me.

There is another way of constructing a relationship beyond suicidal death. One of the common ways in which suicide is constructed in suicide notes is through references to a gift. A person takes their life to make the lives of their significant others better. Consider the following extracts:

**Extract 11**

> I give you freedom you missed so much I wish you much happiness with you friend whom you missed so much and above all with [first name] because you will surely fully renew the acquaintance when you come back. So, you see that I am not such a bad person if I prefer to remove myself rather than kill everybody. Burn my photographs so the son will not have to see me. Why should he be ashamed of me?

**Extract 12**

> I couldn't bear my disability and loneliness, I must go. I do not want to be an old parasite any longer and a stinker. Because I own nothing, I am also a life obstacle for you.

**Extract 13**

> Nothing has worked for me. I lied to you and generally, I have been a bad son. It is better that I am no longer. You will be better off in life, and so will I. I have only been a burden for you.

A gift is always spoken for; it is never free and is always related to an obligation (Mauss, 1990). The act of giving is a form of a contract governed by three major concepts: obligations to give, receive, and repay. The act of giving creates a gift debt that must be repaid, creating a relationship between the giver and receiver.

However, suicide cannot be received and is unlikely to be reciprocated. Indeed, suicide is also unlikely to be intended so. Suicide is an 'inalienable' gift—one that retains a tie to its owner (Weiner, 1992). It is a gift that cannot be disengaged from, and it creates a permanent relationship between the giver and the recipient. Suicide is forever. Thus, the suicide gift makes the relationship with those who are meant to receive it forever. The person who died is there to stay in the lives of those left behind, at least linguistically.

There were, however, a few suicide notes where relationships were constructed with people who were not addressed in the letters. Consider the following note:

**Extract 14**

Everybody will probably blame [first name] for everything. They should all fuck right off because he does not affect me (you are a different matter). When I want, I smoke, when I do not want to, I do not. Recently I smoked, the day before yesterday, and I regret it. Everyone probably thinks that because I was drunk. They cannot be more mistaken. I drank a little bottle for courage, I think I would not have done it sober.

The note is an acknowledgement that a person taking their life continues to be in a relationship with the person who is mentioned but not addressed. It is also an acknowledgement that the act is likely to have consequences for close ones of those who take their lives. The note is an act of preemptive exculpation of the person in question. The note also establishes a close relationship with someone. This time, however, the relationship is that of caring and protecting the person.

We further would like to argue that the following suicide notes can be interpreted similarly:

**Extract 15**

I so wanted, I so did.

**Extract 16**

This is my decision.

**Extract 17**

At the beginning, I would like to point out that what I am doing is my independent decision, although forced by the situation in which I have found myself.

**Extract 18**

I have decided to leave this life. I apologise to you [addressing many].

By emphasising the independence of the suicide decision, the note authors also situate their close ones outside their suicide process. In other words, the authors of the notes above take responsibility for their actions, similar to Extract 14. In addition, the references to the authors' decisions are rendered in unmodalised clauses; there are no qualifications, and no hesitation is even implied. We suggest that there are at least two primary addressees of such notes. On the one hand, it is the close ones who are likely the initial readers of the notes. On the other, the notes are also likely to be addressed to the prosecutors who, by law, are required to investigate every suicidal death.

In this section, we argued that suicide was constructed in relation to a close one. Consistently, references to suicide were made with communicative acts that constructed and underscored the relationships in which the note authors were. Put differently, suicides were not committed because relationships no longer existed; rather, they were committed despite the existing relationships. Moreover, these relationships were constructed to last beyond the suicidal death.

## Agency in Regretting

In this section, we focus on regretting, another kind of account of suicide in which others play an important role. The regretting is consistently related to others. Consider:

**Extract 19**

Only today I realised what kind of mistake I had made. (…) yes, for me it is a great mistake, a great failure because I hurt not only myself but also my children.

**Extract 20**

Today, as I said, I regret a little that I realised that my family suffered because of me. Particularly my son. I now regret that step a little, a little, a little. That I took such action.

**Extract 21**

The first days I spent being observed, I was thinking why they had saved me. And later, when my children started calling me, we started talking and writing to each other, thanks to my children, I understood that I had made a big mistake because they really need me.

**Extract 22**

The children showed me that I am, they said that I am still needed, that I have someone to live for because I have them and a husband. I have grandchildren whom I love greatly. But at that moment, I was not thinking about anyone, only about myself, right?

There are two important aspects of these stories. First, they explicitly construct the speakers as regretting what they did or considering what they did a mistake. Second, and perhaps more significant, such narratives are consistently made with references to the interviewees' families.

Similar to our discussion in the previous section, suicide attempts here are constructed as affecting those close to our informants. The informants do not construct themselves as regretting of their own accord; the regret comes from what their actions did to others. The suicide attempt is not narrated from the perspective of the informant and what they wish for. Rather, their suicide narrative is told from the perspective of another, acknowledging the impact it had on them. The perspective of the speaker sits uneasily alongside that of the family.

The three extracts above show the perspective of regret that adopts the family as its source. It is either a new perspective or one that competes with the previous perspective of the self. In Extract 19, the informant emphasises that the perspective of the family is very new—her realisation happened on the day. Meanwhile, in Extract 20, the informant insists that he regrets a little, underscoring it with the repetition of the phrase. Similarly, in Extract 21, the regret is replaced when the informant starts talking to her family.

The role of the children and a new perspective is emphasised in Extract 22. Not only are they represented as communicators but, we would argue, the informant's story is an account of what the children said. She ends with the rejection of 'thinking about herself', as the close ones' perspective is represented as the appropriate one.

We would like to end this section with two last extracts in which the struggle between regretting the suicide attempt and, at the same time, regretting not having been successful in killing oneself is made explicit. Consider:

**Extract 23**

There are moments when I regret that I was not successful. There are those when I am happy that I was not successful. When I was being

> discharged from (city name), they told me that the decision is truly yours. It is your responsibility whether you kill yourself or will continue living. Well, since we are talking today and I was discharged almost a month ago, I made the right decision, and I am alive.

Although the narrative ends with a declaration of satisfaction with the decision to continue living, the extract directly positions the speaker in two minds about what he should regret. What is significant in this narrative is that the struggle between the two positions is made without reference to the speaker's close ones. It seems that the open ambivalence of the narrative can only be voiced on one's own. Also, the narrative in Extract 24 can only be made without reference to the close ones.

**Extract 24**

> Everything was planned perfectly. I made one tiny mistake, and I cannot come grips with it. I made the mistake that I took the medication drinking alcohol. I forgot that I could lose consciousness at any time. And I was not in control of this. And indeed, I did lose consciousness.

Although there is no reference to regretting not killing herself, the implication of the narrative is quite clear. Just as in Extract 23, the story is told without mentioning the close ones. Families are only spoken about in stories that are meant to be positive.

In this section, we examined the stories of suicidal actions that did not result in the person's death. Two narratives dominated our dataset. First, our informants talked about not understanding what they had done. There were stories of individuals not thinking straight, or having an inability to understand themselves. In those stories, suicide was constructed not as an action performed by an unfettered agent, but as something inexplicable.

The second kind of story focused on regrets of what had happened. What was significant in those stories, however, was that it was not the informants who were the sources of their regrets. Consistently, the regrets were represented as emanating from contacts and explanations from the families.

We discussed the stories of the aftermath of suicide. Consistently, our informants cast their suicidal actions as in relationship with others. It was the relationship, moreover, that resulted in the informants' regrets.

## Conclusions

In this chapter, we discussed the positioning of suicide in relation to those who are left behind after the act. We argued that suicide is consistently portrayed as affecting others. Moreover, and more significantly, we also argued that suicide is described as not affecting the existing relationships. Time and again, writers of suicide notes constructed their relationships as surviving their suicide. Alternatively, our informants in ex-post-facto interviews described their relationships as more important for the future. The regrets they told us about were related to their close ones, who at the same time offered perspectives for the future.

As pointed out at the beginning of the chapter, suicidology is interested in relationships in which a person taking their life finds themselves. However, the dominant suicidological perspective focuses on relationships at the time preceding the suicide. In other words, relationships, or their absence, are either protective or risk factors for people. There is significant research on various relationship configurations and dynamics (e.g., Næss et al., 2021; Stephenson et al., 2023).

In contrast to the dominant suicidological research, we suggest that relationships are important at all stages of the suicide process. In our view, they must not only be perceived as contributing to a set of demographics. Our data suggest that suicidal action is considered not only as resulting from particular relationships but also affecting them. There are a few notes where suicide is not positioned, explicitly or implicitly, as concerning others. The rare research by Oliffe and co-authors (2012) supports the view of relationships as part of the suicide dilemma.

**Extract 25**

I realise that I will hurt many persons, it does not stop bothering me, but one thought has been on my mind all the time. I have already decided, I know I am selfish at this moment, but I beg you, understand, I cannot go on. I would very much like you to understand it and to explain it to my parents. I know it will be a tough nut to crack, but please tell them what happened to me. I know that in this letter, I have not explained anything, but I simply cannot put write it down, let alone say it. It is hard to write at this moment, I am scared a lot, and I am having a brainstorm. Again, I apologise to you, apologise to my parents and do not worry.

An explicit note such as the one above depicts the emotional dilemmas posed by suicides. Once again, such data shows how limited and narrow a view representing suicide is when it is merely described in terms of its upshot. Suicide does not boil down to death, as it is not committed by an individual in a social vacuum.

Our suicide note data also suggests suicide prevention strategies, especially in view of the stories of unending relationships. The common construction of suicide as opening a new life or maintaining the current one must be seen as crucial to address.

Similarly—also for our informants in ex-post-facto interviews—it was relationships that offered narratives of hope for the future. We would like to emphasise, however, that we do not wish to focus on the existence of relationships or their general dynamics. What we are suggesting is that our data offer insight into the lived experiences of individuals who attempted to end their lives and found their relationships enduring.

Once again, such data offer the potential for clinical work with the people after suicide attempts and their close ones. The insight into narrative experiences in such extreme situations can be built on clinical strategies of help and support.

We would also like to offer some commentary on theoretical perspectives on suicide in view of the data we presented here. The first is the issue of intent behind suicide. The consistent depiction of the suicidal person in relationships raises questions about their intent, commitment, and possibilities of stopping the act. As in our discussion of the agency of waiting, also here we see how stories of suicide opens spaces for a better understanding of the process and for prevention.

We also argue that further research is needed on the interactional positions note writers take in their letters. It is significant in our view not only that note authors positioned themselves in a relationship but also what kind of interactional relationship they set up in their letters. For example, notes that were apologies or gifts constructed the writers in different relationships. We think that exploring such relationships can offer further insight into the role of relationships in the suicide process.

Finally, interactional identities also offer insight into how suicide is perceived by those who wrote letters or offered post-attempt narratives. Consistently, people engaging in suicidal action positioned themselves as observers of those they were in a relationship with. While they seemed to ask themselves what their suicide would do to others, they did not seem to ask what the relationship would do to themselves. Indeed, the not-ending-anything suicide suggests that the question of the self in suicide and relationship is absent from the narrative. This, again, seems an important dimension for suicide prevention strategies.

## Note

1 A superordinate clause introduces another clause as, for example, in *He said that he liked me*. The initial superordinate clause (*he said*) tells us how to interpret the other one, the subordinate clause. In other words, the subordinate clause stems from the main one in that it helps narrow down its meaning. In the example given, the subordinate clause narrows down what the saying, referred

to in the superordinate clause, was all about. Coordinate clauses are independent of one another. In a sentence such as *Mary likes me, but Anne doesn't like me.*, the two clauses ('likes' and 'doesn't like') do not depend on each other to make meaning.

## References


Brochu, P. M., Veillette, L. A. S., Serrano, J. M., & Seidl, M. (2021). It's interpersonal: Internalized weight bias and suicidality are associated indirectly via perceived burdensomeness and thwarted belongingness. *Stigma and Health*, *6*(3), 287–295. https://doi.org/10.1037/sah0000264

Carter, S. P., Cobb, E., Novak, L. A., Ekman, E., Ton, A., LaCroix, J. M., & Ghahramanlou-Holloway, M. (2024). The importance of romantic relationships in preventing suicide. *Journal of Family Theory & Review, 16*(2), 352–373. https://doi.org/10.1111/jftr.12559

Cerel, J., Brown, M. M., Maple, M., Singleton, M., Van de Venne, J., Moore, M., & Flaherty, C. (2019). How many people are exposed to suicide? Not six. *Suicide and Life-Threatening Behavior*, *49*(2), 529–534. https://doi.org/10.1111/sltb.12450

Denney, J. T. (2010). Family and household formations and suicide in the United States. *Journal of Marriage and Family*, *72*(1), 202–213. https://doi.org/10.1111/j.1741-3737.2009.00692.x

Eslava, D., Martínez-Vispo, C., Villanueva-Blasco, V. J., Errasti, J. M., & Al-Halabí, S. (2023). Family conflict and suicidal behaviour in adolescence: The mediating role of the assertive interpersonal schema. *Sustainability*, *15*(6), 5149. https://doi.org/10.3390/su15065149

Frey, L. M., & Cerel, J. (2015). Risk for suicide and the role of family: A narrative review. *Journal of Family Issues, 36*(6), 716–736. https://doi.org/10.1177/0192513X13515885

Galasiński, D. (2017). *Discourses of men's suicide notes: A qualitative analysis.* Bloomsbury Publishing.

Joiner, T. E. (2005). *Why people die by suicide.* Harvard University Press.

Kazan, D., Calear, A. L., & Batterham, P. J. (2016). The impact of intimate partner relationships on suicidal thoughts and behaviours: A systematic review. *Journal of Affective Disorders*, *190*, 585–598. https://doi.org/10.1016/j.jad.2015.11.003

Klonsky, E. D., & May, A. M. (2015). The three-step theory (3ST): A new theory of suicide rooted in the 'ideation-to-action' framework. *International Journal of Cognitive Therapy, 8*(2), 114–129. https://doi.org/10.1521/ijct.2015.8.2.114

Mauss, M. (1990). *The gift: The form and reason for exchange in archaic societies.* Routledge.

Næss, E. O., Mehlum, L., & Qin, P. (2021). Marital status and suicide risk: Temporal effect of marital breakdown and contextual difference by socioeconomic status. *SSM – Population Health*, *15*, 100853. https://doi.org/10.1016/j.ssmph.2021.100853

Narita, Z., Shinozaki, T., Goto, A., Hori, H., Kim, Y., Wilcox, H. C., Inoue, M., Tsugane, S., & Sawada, N. (2024). Time-varying living arrangements and suicide death in the general population sample: 14-year causal survival analysis via pooled logistic regression. *Epidemiology and Psychiatric Sciences*, *33*, e30. https://doi.org/10.1017/S2045796024000325

Niu, L., Jia, C., Ma, Z., Wang, G., Sun, B., Zhang, D., & Zhou, L. (2020). Loneliness, hopelessness and suicide in later life: A case-control psychological autopsy study in rural China. *Epidemiology and Psychiatric Sciences*, *29*, e119. https://doi.org/10.1017/S2045796020000335

Oliffe, J. L., Ogrodniczuk, J. S., Bottorff, J. L., Johnson, J. L., & Hoyak, K. (2012). 'You feel like you can't live anymore': Suicide from the perspectives of Canadian men who experience depression. *Social Science & Medicine*, *74*(4), 506–514. https://doi.org/10.1016/j.socscimed.2010.03.057

Purcell, B., Heisel, M. J., Speice, J., Franus, N., Conwell, Y., & Duberstein, P. R. (2012). Family connectedness moderates the association between living alone and suicide ideation in a clinical sample of adults 50 years and older. *The American Journal of Geriatric Psychiatry*, *20*(8), 717–723. https://doi.org/10.1097/JGP.0b013e31822ccd79

Shaw, R. J., Cullen, B., Graham, N., Lyall, D. M., Mackay, D., Okolie, C., Pearsall, R., Ward, J., John, A., & Smith, D. J. (2021). Living alone, loneliness and lack of emotional support as predictors of suicide and self-harm: A nine-year follow up of the UK Biobank cohort. *Journal of Affective Disorders*, *279*, 316–323. https://doi.org/10.1016/j.jad.2020.10.026

Stephenson, M., Prom-Wormley, E., Lannoy, S., & Edwards, A. C. (2023). The temporal relationship between marriage and risk for suicidal ideation. *Journal of Affective Disorders*, *343*, 129–135. https://doi.org/10.1016/j.jad.2023.10.007

Van Orden, K. A., Merrill, K. A., & Joiner, T. E. Jr. (2005). Interpersonal-psychological precursors to suicidal behavior: A theory of attempted and completed suicide. *Current Psychiatry Reviews, 1*(2), 187–196. https://doi.org/10.2174/1573400054065541

Van Orden, K. A., Witte, T. K., Cukrowicz, K. C., Braithwaite, S. R., Selby, E. A., & Joiner, T. E., Jr. (2010). The interpersonal theory of suicide. *Psychological Review*, *117*(2), 575–600. https://doi.org/10.1037/a0018697

Weiner, B. (1992). *Human motivation: Metaphors, theories and research*. Sage.

Wyder, M., Ward, P., & De Leo, D. (2009). Separation as a suicide risk factor. *Journal of Affective Disorders*, *116*(3), 208–213. https://doi.org/10.1016/j.jad.2008.11.007

Yip, P. S., Yousuf, S., Chan, C. H., Yung, T., & Wu, K. C. (2015). The roles of culture and gender in the relationship between divorce and suicide risk: A meta-analysis. *Social Science & Medicine (1982)*, *128*, 87–94. https://doi.org/10.1016/j.socscimed.2014.12.034

Zareian, B., & Klonsky, E. D. (2020). Connectedness and suicide. In A. C. Page & W. G. K. Stritzke (Eds.), *Alternatives to suicide. Beyond risk and toward a life worth living* (pp. 135–158). Academic Press.

## Appendix

### Extract 1

Kocham Was bardzo i przepraszam za to co zrobiłem, ale sytuacja mnie przerosła, nie mogę sobie z tym poradzić wybaczcie mi wszyscy a szczególnie Ty moja kochana [first_name].

### Extract 2

PRZEPRASZAM ZA WSZYSTKO ALE NIE MOGĘ TAK ŻYĆ NERKI BOLĄ NAPRAWDĘ PRZEPRASZAM.

KOCHAM WAS I NAPRAWDĘ PRZEPRASZAM

ŻONO KOCHAM CIĘ.

### Extract 3

Kocham Cię Kocham Cię Kocham Cię Kocham Cię Przepraszam że to co zrobiłem sprawiło Ci ból i rozpacz ale po czasie dojdziesz do wniosku że tak było najlepiej. Zawsze twierdziłem że nie chcę nikogo krzywdzić i dlatego zrobiłem to co zrobiłem.

### Extract 4

Nie wiem czy mi to przebaczysz Ty i dzieci ale proszę Was przebaczcie mi to co Wam zrobiłem żegnajcie

[first_name].

### Extract 5

Przepraszam wszystkich za to co zrobiłem. [first_name] wybacz mi proszę. Kocham Cię bardzo. Nikt nie jest winny tego co się stało.

### Extract 6

Przebacz mi to co zrobiłem i wszystkie krzywdy ode mnie jakie Ci wyrządziłem. Zadzwoń do mej pani doktor [last_name] i powiedz, że ją przepraszam, że ją zawiodłem. Życzę Ci szczęścia beze mnie. Moją córkę [first_name] też przepraszam za to co zrobiłem i za wszystkie krzywdy ode mnie. Przepraszam tych co zawiodłem, wszystkich.

**Extract 7**

Zawsze będę Cię kochał.

**Extract 8**

Kocham Cię i zawsze będziesz w moim sercu.

**Extract 9**

[first_name] będę kochał do końca jej życia

**Extract 10**

kochane moje ja Was bardzo kocham ale już nie mam sił zawsze duchem będę przy Was.

Wybaczcie mi

**Extract 11**

Daję Ci wolność której tak bardzo Ci brakowało życzę Ci dużo szczęścia z Twoimi znajomymi których Ci tak brakowało a przede wszystkim z [first_name] bo pewnie jak wróci dnowisz w 100% waszą znajomość. Także sama widzisz że nie jestem takim złym człowiekiem skoro wolę się usunąć niż wszystkich pozabijać. Popal też moje zdjęcia coby syn nie musiał mnie oglądać po co ma się mnie wstydzić.

**Extract 12**

Nie mogłem dłużej wytrzymać z moim kalectwem i samotnością muszę odejść. Nie chcę być dłużej starym pasożytem i śmierdzielem ponieważ nie posiadam nic a dla Was tylko jestem przeszkodą życiową.

**Extract 13**

Nic mi nie wychodziło. Kłamałem Was i w ogóle byłem złym synem. Lepiej że mnie już nie ma. Lepiej będzie wam żyło i mi. Byłem tylko ciężarem dla Was.

**Extract 14**

Wszyscy pewnie będą obwiniać za wszystko [first_name]. Niech się odpierdolą od niego, bo on nie ma żadnego wpływu na mnie (co innego

Ty). Kiedy chcę to jaram, kiedy nie chcę, to nie. Ostatnio zapaliłem przedwczoraj z nerwów i cholernie żałuję. Wszyscy pewnie myślą, że się powiesiłem dlatego, że byłem pijany. Otóż nic bardziej mylnego. Strzeliłem sobie flaszeczkę na odwagę, bo na trzeźwo bym chyba tego nie zrobił.

**Extract 15**

Tak chciałem i tak zrobiłem

**Extract 16**

To jest moja decyzja

**Extract 17**

Na wstępie chciałbym zaznaczyć, że to co zrobię jest moją samodzielną decyzją, aczkolwiek wymuszoną sytuacją w jakiej się znalazłem.

**Extract 18**

Postanowiłem odejść z tego życia Przepraszam Was.

**Extract 19**

dopiero tutaj zrozumiałam: jaki błąd popełniłam. (...) tak, dla mnie to jest wielki błąd wielka porażka bo skrzywdziłam nie tylko siebie ale i: i: dzieci swoje.

**Extract 20**

dziś tak jak powiedziałem (no) trochę żałuję że po prostu sobie uświadomiłem że po prostu rodzina moja y: ucierpiała przez przez to przeze mnie. syn zwłaszcza i (.) trochę trochę trochę teraz żałuję tego kroku. że tak tak tak postąpiłem.

**Extract 21**

pierwsze dni jak leżałam na obserwacji to myślałam po co mnie uratowali? a później jak już moje dzieci zaczęły do mnie dzwonić zaczęliśmy rozmawiać pisać ze sobą to dzięki dzieciom moim zrozumiałam że zrobiłam duży błąd bo one mnie naprawdę potrzebują.

**Extract 22**

dzieci mi okazały to że ja jestem/ i powiedziały prawda? że ja im jestem jeszcze potrzebna (.) że mam dla kogo żyć i bo mam ich mam męża mam wnuki które strasznie też kocham ale ja wtedy w tym w tym momencie wtedy nie myślałam o nikim tylko o samej sobie prawda?

**Extract 23**

są takie chwile że żałuję że się nie udało. są takie chwile że się cieszę. (.) że się nie udało (.) nie chcę już próbować. (.) gdy wypisywali mnie z [city name] powiedzieli mi decyzja należy tak naprawdę decyzja należy do ciebie. to jest twoja odpowiedzialność. czy się zabijesz czy będziesz żyć. skoro dzisiaj rozmawiamy a wypisano mnie: (.) prawie miesiąc temu (.) to podjąłem właściwą decyzję i żyję.

**Extract 24**

Była dokładnie i <u>moim</u> zdaniem perfekcyjnie zaplanowana. popełniłam tylko jeden maleńki błąd. (.) i: nie mogę się z tym pogodzić. y:m popełniłam taki błąd że zażywając y: leki (.) pijąc alkohol zapomniałam o tym że w każdej chwili mogę stracić świadomość. po prostu nie kontrolowałam tego i: rzeczywiście straciłam świadomość

**Extract 25**

daję sobie sprawę, że bardzo dużo osób skrzywdzę, to mi nie daje spokoju, ale cały czas chodzi mi po głowie jedna myśl. Ja już zdecydowałem, wiem, że jestem w tym momencie egoistą, ale błagam, zrozum, że nie mam już sił, bardzo bym chciał abyś to zrozumiała i wytłumaczyła to moim rodzicom, ja wiem, że będzie to ciężki orzech do zgryzienia, ale bardzo Cię proszę powiedz im co się ze mną stało, wiem, że w tym liście nic nie wytłumaczyłem, ale po prostu nie potrafię tego przelać na papier, ani tym bardziej powiedzieć. Ciężko mi pisać bo w obecnej chwili bardzo się boję, przeżywam burzę mózgu. [...] Jeszcze raz bardzo Cię przepraszam, przeproś ode mnie rodziców, i nie martw się.

# 6 Parents and Suicide

## Introduction

In the previous chapter, we explored the narrated relationships that individuals construct around themselves within the context of suicidal ideation. We also explored how those who took their lives or made serious attempts to do so portrayed themselves within relationships. This was depicted both in the suicide notes, where the narrative preceded the suicidal act and in the post-attempt interviews, where the narrative followed the attempt. In both cases, suicidal individuals focused on others. Our main argument was that suicide is consistently positioned as affecting people. Moreover, and more significantly, we also argued that suicide is portrayed as having a minimal effect on existing relationships. Our analysis revealed that writers of suicide notes frequently constructed their relationships as enduring beyond their suicide.

Suicide is the ultimate method of removing oneself from the family and the wider community (Ratnarajah & Schofield, 2008). Given the enduring emotional bond between a parent and a child, children who experience loss due to the suicide deaths of a parent endure profound and lasting consequences. The quality of the parent–child relationship is crucial for the physical health and psychological well-being of the child. Therefore, the loss of a parent in suicide poses severe risks to the child's future development (Andriessen et al., 2020; Feigelman et al., 2017).

This chapter's aim is to explore discursive constructions of relationships in suicide notes written by parents and explicitly addressed to their children. We are primarily interested in how the writing parent describes the relationship with their child, and also how their relationships with their spouse and other significant people are portrayed.

Our argument is founded on three dominant patterns in the dataset we collected. First, the position taken by the parent is predominantly one of experiencing the world. In the letters, the parents construct themselves as thinking or feeling rather than doing. Second, the addressees of the

DOI: 10.4324/9781032672847-6

letters are constructed in two ways. On the one hand, they are explicitly positioned in a relationship with the writing parent and have a negative impact on the parent; on the other, they are described in positive terms. Third, the few letters that refer to third parties consistently describe them in negative terms.

## Being a Parent

Parental responsibilities have evolved significantly throughout history, from focusing on basic needs, safety, and guiding children's moral and ethical development, to encompassing a broader range of tasks, including education, emotional support, and socialisation (Lamb, 2000; Cunningham, 2020). Mothers' roles have been associated with caring and nurturing, while fathers have been portrayed as emotionally unavailable breadwinners (Finn & Henwood, 2009; Johansson, 2011). For example, Gaunt and Scott's study (2017) found that following the arrival of a child, a woman's parental role becomes higher in the role hierarchy, displacing the professional role. For men, the arrival of a child is associated with an increase in the importance of professional activity. However, there has been a gradual shift from traditional gender roles with the promotion of a caring father (Hunter et al., 2017), as well as women's increased participation in the workforce (Latshaw & Hale, 2015).

The ideological landscape of fatherhood is more complicated. The ever stronger pressure to provide is firmly coupled with women's claims to the traditionally masculine spheres of life (Featherstone, 2009; Miller, 2011). Zoja (2001) posits that fatherhood is ridden by a paradox of opposing roles a father has. The father's 'success' is measured on the one hand by his interaction with the child, but also, crucially, by how he interacts with society. To make things more complicated, Zoja adds that the children themselves want the father to succeed in the world; they want him to be strong and victorious. There are unprecedented levels of absent fathers from families (Coltrane (2004) quoted in Dermott, 2008) coupled with increasing pressure for 'new fatherhood' as an emotional involvement with the child (O'Brien, 2005). While researchers talk about fatherhood and its various configurations (Miller, 2011), they get away from a unified model of masculinity and/or fatherhood (Vuori, 2009). Indeed, fatherhood is more precarious and insecure, as the father, who gives more and more, matters less and less (Zoja, 2001).

### *Suicide of a Parent*

Although research suggests that parenthood is associated with a lower risk of suicide (Dehara et al., 2021; Denney, 2010; Høyer & Lund, 1993), it is estimated that between 7,000 and 30,000 children in the United States experience a parent's suicide each year (Cerel et al., 2008; Hung & Rabin, 2009).

The protective nature of parenthood appears to be particularly relevant for women. According to Krüger and co-authors (2017), mothers gain more protection from having children than fathers. This is seconded by Qin and Mortensen (2003) who argue that having a young child has a much stronger influence on women than on men. For men, the protective effect of having children was significant only when having a child from birth to age one, whereas, for women, it was significant until the child reached the age of 18 (see also: Weisenhorn et al., 2017). However, there have also been emerging data showing that suicide is a leading cause of death in the perinatal period, accounting for about 20% of postpartum deaths (Chin et al., 2022; Trost et al., 2021; Biggs et al., 2023). On the other hand, parents of children with a hospitalised psychiatric disorder, and parents of children who have died are at an increased risk of suicide (Qin & Mortensen, 2003).

Frey and Cerel (2015) argue that researchers have failed to address whether parenthood influences parents who commit suicide. It remains unclear whether the protective effect of parenthood on suicide risk is due to differences in the factors that influence the decision to become a parent or to remain childless. For example, physically and mentally healthy people are more likely to have children. The question then arises as to the extent these factors (e.g., being healthy) are responsible for the protective nature of parenthood and to the extent that having children is protective (Dahera et al., 2021). Therefore, a possible explanation for the parenting effect, according to Dahera and co-authors (2021), is that having children may expand parents' social connectedness by enabling them to meet other parents and acquaintances through their children, thus reducing loneliness. The presence of more than one child may further enhance the sense of belonging and support, as well as social connectedness, by increasing interactions with other adults in the children's environment. Finally, the lower suicide risk observed among parents with at least two children may be partly due to greater relationship stability, as couples who separate after having one child are less likely to have additional children.

The Interpersonal Theory of Suicide (ITS) proposes that children can also be seen as alleviating loneliness, thereby reducing feelings of thwarted belonging (Joiner, 2005; Van Orden et al., 2005; Van Orden et al., 2010). Children give parents a greater sense of purpose and direction in life, instilling a sense of obligation, responsibility, and caring to increase feelings of belonging. This, in turn, can reduce suicidal ideation and behaviours (Sörberg Wallin et al., 2022). On the other hand, Cerel (2006 cited in Fray & Cerel, 2015) found that conflict with children or a spouse regarding the former often preceded a suicide attempt by adults who were parents. Overall, conflict and difficulties in romantic relationships significantly increase the risk of suicide (Boardman et al., 1999; Duberstein et al., 2004). Unfortunately, as Frey and Cerel (2015), and Zareian and Klonsky (2020) argue, there is limited research on how the quality of the parent–child relationship affects the risk of parental suicide. More research is needed to better understand the protective role of parenting against suicide.

In this chapter, we focus only on suicide letters. This is because we are interested in messages addressed explicitly to surviving children. Only suicide letters offer this kind of channel of communication. We selected letters that are explicitly addressed to the children of the letter writer. The letters we included in our dataset had at least one of the following characteristics:

- The addressees were explicitly addressed as children, either in the salutation (e.g., 'Dear children'), or in the body of the letter (e.g. 'I am writing to you, my son').
- The letters explicitly identified the author of the letter as a parent, either in the body of the letter (e.g., 'forgive me, your father') or in the signature (e.g., 'your mum').

The above parameters were the only way in which we could identify the writing parents. We realise, therefore, that there might be letters written by a parent to their child that we did not include in the dataset. Altogether, we included 42 such letters (22 from mothers and 20 from fathers) in the dataset to be discussed in this chapter.

In our analyses we focused on three linguistically constructed subject positions; they are clauses:

- referring to the speaking parent, through self-reference rendered by the first person singular[1] or plural;
- referring to the addressee; in the dataset at hand, they are the writers' children, with the use of the second person singular or plural;
- referring to others in the third person singular or plural.

## I, the Parent

The writing parents construct themselves predominantly with the use of mental processes (Halliday, 1994). That is to say, they use verbs that refer to mental activity, for example, thinking, considering, and feeling. We would like to start our discussion with a longer letter rendering well the dataset we have.

**Extract 1**

I do not know whether you will ever be able to understand my action and forgive me. In any case, I am not asking for forgiveness, I have no right. You two and Dad have been the greatest treasures of my life. You three has been the goal, happiness, love, all that is most beautiful. At the time when one of you were missing, a link in the chain, my world has collapsed. I have not been able to get up. I tried for a long time but each day was worse than the previous one. I tried so hard to put everything in order anew. And I could not. I suffered so much that I cannot describe it. You were not able to help me. You are young and have a right to life and happiness. Your life is still ahead of you. Many bad and good moments await you. I am not afraid for you. You are clever and will manage. I could not. I had no right to burden you with my suffering. I did not want you to look as I fight the windmills. For two and a half years I have tried to live. I did not manage. I regret nothing. I loved you Dad over anything else in the world. Over my own life.

The writing parent's story mostly uses mental processes, with verbs such as 'know', 'fear', 'suffer', and 'want'. In addition, references to mental states are done implicitly with phrases such as 'you were the treasure', 'you were direction, happiness, love', and 'fighting windmills'. The writing mother describes the world through her perspective. This includes loss and bereavement, and the relationships in the family. The perspectives of the addressees of the letter—the author's children—are absent from the account.

This is typical of the dataset we have. Consider also the following fragments in which the first two extracts (Extract 2–3) come from mothers, and the remaining two come from fathers (Extract 4–5):

**Extract 2**

I admire you. That despite my unpleasant, depressing behaviour, you attain very good results. I dreamt so much as about your final exam results, that I will be watching your successes at work.

**Extract 3**

I love you so much and I miss you. I cannot bear all this, it is difficult, I am tired of living.

**Extract 4**

I love you and it is most difficult to leave because I cannot see you at the end. I looked at your picture for two days and I wept with happiness that I have such a wonderful son. Your forever loving you dad.

**Extract 5**

I wanted the best for you.

What is striking in the extracts above is that they primarily focus on the writing parents. Even when constructing a relationship between the parent and the child addressed in the notes, the child is represented as an object of the parent's actions. And it is these actions that are the main topic of the notes. Moreover, the parents' self-reference in terms of mental activities makes the notes confessional. They are the parent's last words, either expressing positive emotions for the children or, in a minority of cases, expressing suffering. The relationship between the parent and the child is constructed almost exclusively in terms of positive emotions, such as love, longing, or wanting the best for the child.

However, occasionally, the parent constructs themselves in negative terms. Consider:

**Extract 6**

Dear children, forgive me what bad I did to you. I love you and forgive me that I have failed you. I love you. I cannot live like that any longer. I leave you [a small sum of money]. It will be enough for taxes national insurance. Again, I love you all, stay with God and be healthy.

**Extract 7**

I loved life very much and what I did was for you. But that nightmarish pain is no longer bearable. It is in every bit of my body. I cannot destroy you anymore. Forgive me, I have no more strength to fight even though I would so much like to be with you. I love you very much but you must live on.

**Extract 8**

I cannot bear the tinnitus in my ears and the pills. Mum.
I was good for nothing anyway.

The negative constructions are not direct, though. In Extract 6, the writing father introduces the statement about failing into a presupposition (an implied statement that is necessary for the sentence to make sense). In other words, the author of the note does not make a direct claim that he had failed his children but only asks them to forgive the failing. In Extract 7, the writing mother references destroying the children. Her claim is not so much that she destroys them, but that she mustn't do it; the reference to destroying is, again, presupposed.

Extract 8, finally, is the least direct reference to negativity in relationships. In part, it is rendered by the ambiguity of 'I was good for nothing', which, in the context, can mean that the person found it difficult to live, or that others found her difficult to live with. Such ambiguity presumably softens the message about the nature of the person's relationships.

The final point we would like to make about the parents' self-reference in the notes is that the positivity of their relationship with their children does not end with their death. Consider the following extracts:

**Extract 9**

My little daughters, I will always be by your side. I love you and do not be sad. I will be free at last. [...] My dearest I love you very much, but I have no more strength. I will be by your side in spirit.

**Extract 10**

[First name] forgive me that I have failed you, but I can see that you are fading away. The longer I am here, the more I destroy you. And you must live for the children. I have no physical chance. I love you very much and I will love you.

**Extract 11**

I love you very much and I will love you at every moment even if I am no longer there. Forgive me that I have taken your joy and youth away. That I have inflicted so much unpleasantness on you.

**Extract 12**

I am sorry I will not be at your first communion when you go to school and I will not be able to see how you grow up. I want you to know that I love you very much and that part of me will always be by your side.

The notes are uniform in promising love and presence beyond suicide as if the act were not putting an end to the person's life and, in the process, their feelings. Crucially, the fragments refer to the feelings that the authors of the letters will continue to have. In Extract 9, the father promises to be with them, whereas in Extracts 10 and 11, the mothers say they will love their children. All three fragments are constructed in active voice, placing the writer as the actor.

Significantly, the mother in Extract 11 makes it clear that she will love the children, even in her absence. It is as if she wants to make sure that she understands that the promise is somewhat out of the ordinary. We propose that this is a strategy for making the promise more realistic and acceptable. Similarly, we think that the reference to being there 'in spirit' in Extract 9 and to 'a part of me' in Extract 12, have a similar function. The phrases make them more suited to the promises after the parent's death.

In this section, we discussed how parents construct themselves in their suicide notes. The dataset suggests that the notes are used confessionally, that is to say, the writing parents focus predominantly on themselves and their feelings. Recasting the practice of recording oneself visually, one could say that the letters are the final written 'selfie' of the parents. As the parents confess their love and promise their presence, often everlasting, they seem to offer the final word of encouragement or support. The child could always go back to the note and find succour in it.

## You, the Child

In this section, we move to discuss how the addressees (the children) of parental suicide notes are constructed. In contrast to the mostly positive picture of the parents painted in the notes, their children are represented in a more ambivalent way. There are two main ways in which such representations are made in the letters. On the one hand, when the children are described on their own, they are consistently shown in positive terms. On the other hand, however, when they are placed in a relationship with the writing parent, they are described in negative terms. We shall discuss them in turn.

Consider the following examples:

### Extract 13

You three are the only and biggest love of my life. You have been my dearest treasures. I will always be by your side. You will always feel my presence. I know you will be happy.

**Extract 14**

> My dearest children son [names] and [name] take care of yourselves [names]. My dearest grandchildren [names], I am very proud of you. That you are so wonderful, you do not complain. Take care of yourselves in the future, of health and love. Go to church and pray.

**Extract 15**

> I love you and it is most difficult to leave because I cannot see you at the end. I looked at your picture for two days and I wept with happiness that I have such a wonderful son. Your forever loving you dad.

**Extract 16**

> Take care of mummy and be good. And above all do not listen to grandmom [first name] because she is dim and can only destroy people. Learn diligently and do what you feel, go after your goals. You are a wonderful guy, and everything is possible for you.

The final words from the parent are those of positivity and praise. Notably, the accounts of the children are constructed from the parent's perspective. The children are not represented as good, clever, or the like in their own right, but the parent endows those characteristics upon them. Put differently, references to children are consistently introduced through superordinate clauses in which the parent refers to their own experience. In the process, we only get to hear about what the parent feels or thinks about their child.

In Extract 13, the children are represented as the mother's greatest love and treasure. In Extract 14, we learn about the positive characteristics through the superordinate clause referring to the mother's pride. Similarly, Extract 15 refers to the parent's crying out of happiness through which the reference to the wonderful son is introduced. Extract 16, however, is different. The note contains advice for the son on how to behave in the future. The writing father offers instructions on who to obey and how to proceed in life. His final words ('you are a wonderful guy…') do not seem much like simple praise but justification for the advice.

The perspective through which to see the children is continued in notes where there is no obvious account of the children. Many notes continue to confess parental love in our dataset, and there are as many confessions as there are constructions of a particular relationship with the addressee (see also Fincham et al., 2011), the 'loved person'. The notes make claims about both the action of the parent who is about to take their life and the social position of the addressees. Consider:

**Extract 17**

[Names] – I love you.

**Extract 18**

My beloved little son, do not be angry that I am leaving. I love you. Your mother.

**Extract 19**

My kids, [names] I love you.

**Extract 20**

I have loved only you.

**Extract 21**

[first name]. I love you more than my life. I am leaving because of your mum. [first name]. I love you very much.

The extracts above are a spectrum of confessional notes in which an expression of love is a central part. Extract 21 seems to convey the kind of message that juxtaposes two persons: the child's mother and the child. The constructed opposition is between good and evil, that is, the mother who is the reason for suicide, and the child who is loved. Extract 20 is quite similar; it constructs the addressee as the only person whom the suicidal parent loved.

We discussed the representation of the addressees of the parental suicide notes. We examined the notes in which the children are constructed consistently in positive terms. However, we only see the child through the parent's perspective. In other words, we primarily learn about the children through their parent's confessions. This is how we also see frequent notes in which the writing parent expresses their love for the child. It is not only that the parent loves the child, but the child is also loved, and deserving of that love.

In the next section, we move to discuss how parental suicide notes represent relationships with the children. In contrast to the mostly positive picture of the children, these relationships are represented more negatively. Some of the notes cross over to being aggressive.

*Relationships*

The confessional notes expressing parental love construct the writing parent as positively contributing to the relationship with their child/children. In this section, however, we discuss how the children's contribution is constructed. There are two points we would like to make here. First, the children are consistently described in negative terms; they are presented as toxic in the relationship. Second, it is the parents' perspective that is consistently invoked in the judging of the children. Consider the following examples:

**Extract 22**

[First name] I know you hate me but I want you to know that I have acted this way because my nerves could not bear it.

**Extract 23**

One more thing, I hope you are pleased now. You will no longer drive me out of the house.

**Extract 24**

[First name]. I saw you at the cemetery, but you did not come up to me. I think you were ashamed of me. Father.

**Extract 25**

Despite that, you do not like me much but I know who is urging you [to be like that]. Do not be so gobby as your mum because you will have it hard in life. After all, you were fond of me but suddenly, bosh, she has taught you to go round the courts and the police. I wish you to be healthy your entire life, to finish all school you will choose. And when you get married consider it well. I give you my blessing right now.[2]

The notes portray the children as hating the parent (Extract 22), chasing them out of the house (Extract 23), in some cases, being ashamed of the father (Extract 24), and simply not liking the parent (Extract 25). In all four examples, the negative description is introduced via the parent's perspective. The writing parents again refer to knowing, hoping, or seeing the children's behaviour. Similar to the previous group of notes in the earlier section, it is their perspective that is invoked in judgement.

Extract 25 is particularly interesting here. The negative assessment of the daughter is softened by the ascription of blame to a third person, presumably the girl's mother. This is where the invocation of the father's perspective happens. While his assessment is hedged with the phrase 'too much', which introduces a perspective through which the statement is made, the reference to the external source of negativity is upping the ante; it is explicit and stresses certainty. In contrast, the negativity with which the girl is described is juxtaposed with the father's good wishes. In such a way, the note also serves the function of a fond farewell, a note the child could come back to.

We end this discussion with three notes that are unusual given the samples of the dataset we have analysed so far. Let us first discuss probably the most aggressive of the notes:

**Extract 26**

Out of the house you whore, you unneeded bitch, you fucked around. Take all that is yours and get the fuck out.[3]

The rudeness of the note is striking; very few notes in the entire corpus are so rude. In the subset of the corpus we analyse here, it is the only note that can be considered rude. The rudeness is used to underscore the message of utter negativity. The daughter is called a whore and a bitch who fucked around. There is no doubt that any competent language user would understand that this note is attempting to offend, and hurt the addressee. This letter does not only express emotions, but it is also aimed at hurting the addressee.

However, linguistically, the note is in the imperative mood; it is a command. The addressee is told to 'get the fuck out', going beyond the writing person's presence. The command is aimed at arranging life after the note author's death as if they had the power to make such a demand.

In the next note, the writing father constructs his daughter as guilty of his death:

**Extract 27**

[First name] you know very well why I have done it. If you have doubts, ask your mummy. I am only your father and have loved you very much. But mum has wrecked my life. She wanted to live wealthily, and she was successful in this. She has always dreamed of a rich life. But you as my daughter will have me on your conscience till the end of your life. And do not think that I was so stupid that your mum arranged a trip to

> [country] for me. I understood everything, the children I loved so much betrayed me very much.

The blame for suicide is implied. The reference to the daughter having the father on her conscience is ambiguous and does not explicitly apportion blame. However, the phrase 'have someone on one's conscience' refers clearly to a person's death. The statement is augmented by the adverbial 'till the end of your life'.

The note is interesting also because it changes the perspective from which it is written. The author starts by addressing his daughter but ends with a third-person account of the children who betrayed their father. The shift in the grammatical form suggests changing the account to a more 'objective' one; the narrator tells it 'like it is', rather than recounting their experience. The last sentence juxtaposes the expression of fatherly love with an 'objective' betrayal, thus making the betrayal crueller. The objectivity of the last sentence can also be perceived as serving as evidence for the preceding harsh words of blame. In other words, this is not just a story invented by the father; the guilt-tripping has a foundation in facts.

What is striking in the account, however, is that in contrast to the preponderance of parental suicide notes, this one not only says something negative about a child to whom the note is addressed; it is also an act of blaming. The confessional note is not an attempt to help the child cope with the parent's suicide—it is the opposite. The note seems aimed at making the child's life worse after the parent's suicide.

The final note in this chapter is also unique in the dataset we have. Consider:

**Extract 30**

> Also, remember that you are to hate your father [full name] because he has never had any respect for me and will never have it for you.

The fragment is a reversal of those we have just discussed. Earlier, the parent complained about being disliked or hated, but, in this case, the mother writing the note demands hate from the child. The note reaches out into the future but, this time, it aims to set up the relationship between the mother's children and their father.

As in Extract 27, the writing mother offers a rationale for her demand—the father's lack of respect for her. She also predicts the future by declaring that the lack of respect will continue although it will be directed at the addressees of the note. It is difficult to see the message only in confessional terms. The note sets out to influence the future of the children and affect their relationship with their father. The mother seems to take revenge on her children's father from behind her grave.

## Conclusion

In this chapter, we examined suicide notes that were written by parents on the precipice of taking their lives. They were addressed to their surviving children. We were interested in exploring discursive constructions of relationships in such notes. Parents in their letters to their children were mostly represented as experiencing the world. Their confessional letters told the addressees about what the letter authors thought or felt. When they wrote about the children, it was also done through the parent's perspective. Consistently, it was the parent who linguistically endowed the child with their positive characteristics. The last kind of notes focused on parents who wrote about what their children did to them. Such notes consistently represented the children in a negative light.

Suicidology commonly assumes that suicide notes are 'ultrapersonal', as was stressed by Leenaars (2004). It leads researchers to assume that suicide notes are a window into the minds of those about to take their lives. However, the notes we discussed in this chapter challenge such assumptions. The notes we quote here have addressees. They are written to be read, often with an explicit addressee. Such notes cannot be seen as written for their own sake and never to be found. The notes for the children are likely intended to settle accounts—make the last statement.

Suicide notes must be understood as semi-public texts. They are more than likely to be read in institutional contexts and by people they are not addressed to. The suicide notes under analysis suggest that their authors were likely to be aware of it. Moreover, the direct addressees are unlikely to be the only ones. It is very likely that other, unlicensed (i.e., not intended to read the note; Clark & Carlson, 1982) readers are assumed to have access to the notes. This, in turn, changes the nature of communication in a suicide note. If an individual knows that someone is likely to read their communication, they make sure to write what can or indeed should be read by additional recipients.

The second issue is the practically non-existent research into suicide notes' reception. This, again, we suspect arises from the assumption of ultra-confidentiality of the notes and their alleged insight into the mind of the writer. However, as they are directed at people, understanding how they are received, and the social and psychological meanings, is crucial in understanding the social nature of suicide and suicide communication.

More importantly, a suicide letter is a fragment of communication that never was. A suicide letter opens a channel of communication only to close it immediately. The meaning of such a message and the fact that it cannot be responded to surely offers useful perspectives on suicide. Such research, moreover, is not only of academic significance. Its results could strongly underpin clinical perspectives on the work with children bereaved by suicide.

Finally, the data we analysed offer important insights into suicide contexts, especially from the viewpoint of the person who takes their life. Incidentally, such data offer valuable perspectives on suicidology. Social scientific research in to parenthood, childhood, and family relations could also benefit from analysing parental suicide letters.

In the following chapter, we continue to focus on stories of parents who took their lives with particular interest in the parent's legacy—the impact of the deceased parent on the surviving child and their life.

## Notes

1 In contrast to English, Polish is a pro-drop language. This means that some pronouns (including *ja*/*my* ('I'/'we') and *ty*/wy ('you', both singular and plural) can be omitted from the linguistic form of the clause. In such cases, the grammatical person of the clause is rendered by the form of the verb in the clause predicate. This is why we prefer to speak of the grammatical person (i.e., the linguistic reference to the event participant, typically, the speaker, the addressee, others) rather than the pronouns themselves.

2 Two comments on the translation are needed. First, the phrase 'you were fond of me' is a translation of Polish *byłaś za mną*. The literal meaning of the phrase is 'you were for me/behind me', which is a regional way of expressing fondness or liking. There is no obvious idiomatic equivalent in English. The second issue is 'after all', which is how we rendered Polish *przecież*, and has no English equivalent. It is a participle introducing a statement polemical with what was said before and one that is obvious to the speaker.

3 The note contains a word that neither of us is familiar with. The verb 'tichać' does not appear in the dictionaries of the Polish language. There are two possibilities. First, the word might be used exclusively in a dialect/sociolect and is not recorded in dictionaries of representing the notional all-Poland language. This might particularly be the case if the word is considered vulgar. Second, there might have been an error in the scanning of the word from the original hand-written note (to which we have no access). As the word does not appear in the national corpus of Polish (www.nkjp.uni.lodz.pl/), the second possibility seems more likely.

## References


Andriessen, K., Krysinska, K., Rickwood, D., & Pirkis, J. (2020). 'It Changes Your Orbit': The impact of suicide and traumatic death on adolescents as experienced by adolescents and parents. *International Journal of Environmental Research and Public Health*, *17*(24), 9356. https://doi.org/10.3390/ijerph17249356

Biggs, L. J., Jephcott, B., Vanderwiel, K., Melgaard, I., Bott, S., Paderes, M., Borninkhof, J., & Birks, M. (2023). Pathways, contexts, and voices of shame and compassion: A grounded theory of the evolution of perinatal suicidality. *Qualitative Health Research*, *33*(6), 521–530. https://doi.org/10.1177/10497323231164278

Boardman, A. P., Grimbaldeston, A. H., Handley, C., Jones, P. W., & Willmott, S. (1999). The North Staffordshire Suicide Study: A case-control study of suicide in one health district. *Psychological Medicine*, *29*(1), 27–33. https://doi.org/10.1017/s0033291798007430

Cerel, J. (2006, April). Suicide attempts in parents of minor children. *Paper presented at the Annual Conference of the American Association of Suicidology*, Seattle, WA.

Cerel, J., Jordan, J. R., & Duberstein, P. R. (2008). The impact of suicide on the family. *Crisis: The Journal of Crisis Intervention and Suicide Prevention, 29*(1), 38–44. https://doi.org/10.1027/0227-5910.29.1.38

Chin, K., Wendt, A., Bennett, I. M., & Bhat, A. (2022). Suicide and maternal mortality. *Current Psychiatry Reports*, *24*(4), 239–275. https://doi.org/10.1007/s11920-022-01334-3

Clark, H. H. & Carlson, T. (1982). Hearers and speech acts. *Language*, *58*, 332–373.

Coltrane, S. (2004). Fathering: Paradoxes, contradictions, and dilemmas. In M. Coleman & L. Ganong (Eds.), *Handbook of contemporary families* (pp. 224–243). Sage.

Cunningham, H. (2020). *Children and childhood in Western society since 1500*. Routledge.

Dehara, M., Wells, M. B., Sjöqvist, H., Kosidou, K., Dalman, C., & Sörberg Wallin, A. (2021). Parenthood is associated with lower suicide risk: A register-based cohort study of 1.5 million Swedes. *Acta Psychiatrica Scandinavica*, *143*(3), 206–215. https://doi.org/10.1111/acps.13240

Denney, J. T. (2010). Family and household formations and suicide in the United States. *Journal of Marriage and Family*, *72*(1), 202–213. https://doi.org/10.1111/j.1741-3737.2009.00692.x

Dermott, E. (2008). *Intimate fatherhood*. Routledge.

Duberstein, P. R., Conwell, Y., Conner, K. R., Eberly, S., & Caine, E. D. (2004). Suicide at 50 years of age and older: Perceived physical illness, family discord and financial strain. *Psychological Medicine*, *34*(1), 137–146. https://doi.org/10.1017/s0033291703008584

Featherstone, B. (2009). *Contemporary fathering: Theory, policy and practice*. Policy Press.

Feigelman, W., Rosen, Z., Joiner, T., Silva, C., & Mueller, A. S. (2017). Examining longer-term effects of parental death in adolescents and young adults: Evidence from the national longitudinal survey of adolescent to adult health. *Death Studies*, *41*(3), 133–143. https://doi.org/10.1080/07481187.2016.1226990

Fincham, B., Langer, S., Scourfield, J., & Shiner, M. (2011). *Understanding suicide: A social autopsy*. Palgrave Macmillan.

Finn, M., & Henwood, K. (2009). Exploring masculinities within men's identificatory imaginings of first-time fatherhood. *British Journal of Social Psychology*, *48*(3), 547–562. https://doi.org/10.1348/014466608X386099

Frey, L. M., & Cerel, J. (2015). Risk for suicide and the role of family: A narrative review. *Journal of Family Issues, 36*(6), 716–736. https://doi.org/10.1177/0192513X13515885

Gaunt, R., & Scott, J. (2017). Gender differences in identities and their sociostructural correlates: How gendered lives shape parental and work identities. *Journal of Family Issues, 38*(13), 1852–1877. https://doi.org/10.1177/0192513X16629182

Halliday, M. A. K. (1994). *An introduction to functional grammar* (2nd ed.). Edward Arnold.

Høyer, G., & Lund, E. (1993). Suicide among women related to number of children in marriage. *Archives of General Psychiatry*, *50*(2), 134–137. https://doi.org/10.1001/archpsyc.1993.01820140060006

Hung, N. C., & Rabin, L. A. (2009). Comprehending childhood bereavement by parental suicide: A critical review of research on outcomes, grief processes, and interventions. *Death Studies*, *33*(9), 781–814. https://doi.org/10.1080/07481180903142357

Hunter, S. C., Riggs, D. W., & Augoustinos, M. (2017). Hegemonic masculinity versus a caring masculinity: Implications for understanding primary caregiving fathers. *Social and Personality Psychology Compass, 11*(3), e12307. https://doi.org/10.1111/spc3.12307

Johansson, T. (2011). The conundrum of fatherhood. Theoretical explorations. *International Journal of Sociology of the Family*, *37*(2), 227–242.

Joiner, T. E. (2005). *Why people die by suicide*. Harvard University Press.

Krüger, S., Priebe, S., Fritsch, R., & Mundt, A. P. (2017). Burden of separation and suicide risk of prisoners with minor children. *International Journal of Law and Psychiatry, 52*, 55–61. https://doi.org/10.1016/j.ijlp.2017.03.004

Lamb, M. E. (2000). The history of research on father involvement: An overview. *Marriage & Family Review*, *29*(2-3), 23–42. https://doi.org/10.1300/J002v29n02_03

Latshaw, B. A., & Hale, S. I. (2015). 'The domestic handoff': Stay-at-home fathers' time-use in female breadwinner families. *Journal of Family Studies*, *22*(2), 97–120. https://doi.org/10.1080/13229400.2015.1034157

Leenaars, A. A. (2004). *Psychotherapy with suicidal people*. Wiley.

Miller, T. (2011). *Making sense of fatherhood: Gender, caring and work*. Cambridge University Press.

O'Brien, M. (2005). *Shared caring: Bringing fathers into the frame*. EOC.

Qin, P., & Mortensen, P. B. (2003). The impact of parental status on the risk of completed suicide. *Archives of General Psychiatry*, *60*(8), 797–802. https://doi.org/10.1001/archpsyc.60.8.797

Ratnarajah, D., & Schofield, M. J. (2008). Survivors' narratives of the impact of parental suicide. *Suicide and Life-Threatening Behavior*, *38*(5), 618–630. https://doi.org/10.1521/suli.2008.38.5.618

Sörberg Wallin, A., Sjöqvist, H., Dehara, M., Wells, M. B., Dykxhoorn, J., Kosidou, K., & Dalman, C. (2022). Parenthood and lower risk of suicide in women and men: The total Swedish population followed across adulthood. *Social Psychiatry and Psychiatric Epidemiology*, *57*(11), 2241–2250. https://doi.org/10.1007/s00127-022-02321-y

Trost, S. L., Beauregard, J. L., Smoots, A. N., Ko, J. Y., Haight, S. C., Moore Simas, T. A., Byatt, N., Madni, S. A., & Goodman, D. (2021). Preventing pregnancy-related mental health deaths: Insights from 14 US Maternal Mortality Review Committees, 2008-17. *Health Affairs (Project Hope)*, *40*(10), 1551–1559. https://doi.org/10.1377/hlthaff.2021.00615

Van Orden, K. A., Merrill, K. A., & Joiner, T. E., Jr. (2005). Interpersonal-psychological precursors to suicidal behavior: A theory of attempted and completed suicide. *Current Psychiatry Reviews, 1*(2), 187–196. https://doi.org/10.2174/1573400054065541

Van Orden, K. A., Witte, T. K., Cukrowicz, K. C., Braithwaite, S. R., Selby, E. A., & Joiner, T. E., Jr. (2010). The interpersonal theory of suicide. *Psychological Review*, *117*(2), 575–600. https://doi.org/10.1037/a0018697

Vuori, J. (2009). Men's choices and masculine duties. Fathers in expert discussions. *Men and Masculinities*, *12*(1), 45–72. https://doi.org/10.1177/1097184X07306720

Weisenhorn, D. A., Frey, L. M., Hans, J. D., & Cerel, J. (2017). Suicide ideation, anxiety, and depression: Are children a protective factor for male Veterans? *Journal of Family Social Work*, *20*(1), 41–51. https://doi.org/10.1080/10522158.2017.1286278

Zareian, B., & Klonsky, E. D. (2020). Connectedness and suicide. In A.C. Page & W. G. K. Stritzke (Eds.), *Alternatives to suicide. Beyond risk and toward a life worth living* (pp. 135–158). Academic Press.

Zoja, L. (2001). *Father*. Brunner-Routledge.

## Appendix

### Extract 1

Nie wiem czy kiedykolwiek będziecie w stanie zrozumieć mój czyn i wybaczyć mi. Zresztą nie proszę o wybaczenie, nie mam prawa. Wy obie i Tata *byliście największymi skarbami mojego życia*. Wasza trójka *stanowiła mój cel, szczęście, miłość, wszystko co najpiękniejsze*. W momencie kiedy zabrakło jednego z Was, jednego ogniwa w tym łańcuszku zawalił się świat. Nie potrafiłam się podnieść. Próbowałam bardzo długo ale każdy dzień był gorszy od poprzedniego. Tak się starałam poukładać wszystko od nowa. I nie mogłam. Cierpiałam tak strasznie, że nie umiem tego opisać. Wy nie byłyście w stanie mi pomóc. Jesteście młode, macie pełne prawo do życia i szczęścia. Wasze życie dopiero przed Wami. Czeka Was dużo złych i dobrych chwil. Nie boję się o Was. Jesteście mądre i dacie sobie radę. Ja nie umiałam. Nie miałam prawa obarczać Was moim cierpieniem. Nie chciałam żebyście patrzyły jak walczę z wiatrakami. Przez dwa i pół roku starałam się żyć, nie udało mi się. Niczego nie żałuję. Kochałam Waszego Tatę i Was ponad wszystko na świecie, ponad własne życie.

**Extract 2**

Podziwiam Was, że mimo mojego przykrego, przygnębiającego zachowania osiągacie bardzo dobre wyniki. Tak bardzo marzyłam, że będę na absolutoriach, będę patrzeć jak osiągacie wyniki w pracy.

**Extract 3**

Kocham Was tak bardzo i tęsknię. Nie zniosę tego wszystkiego, to trudne, jestem zmęczona życiem.

**Extract 4**

Kocham Cię i najtrudniej mi odejść bo nie mogę Cię nawet na koniec zobaczyć dwa dni patrzyłem na Twoje zdjęcie i płakałem ze szczęścia że mam tak cudownego syna.

Twój zawsze kochający Cię tata

**Extract 5**

CHCIAŁEM DLA WAS JAK NAJLEPIEJ

**Extract 6**

Kochane Dzieci wybaczcie mi co złego wam zrobiłem ja was kocham i wybaczcie mi że Was zawiodłem. ja was kocham. ja nie mogę tak dłużej żyć zostawiam wam sześćset czterdzieści złotych. urządzi ma trochę pieniędzy a reszta zlozu i zusu. Jeszcze raz kocham was wszystkich zostańcie Bogiem i bądźcie zdrowi

**Extract 7**

Bardzo kochałam życie i to co robiłam dla Was ale ten ból potworny jest już nie do zniesienia jest w każdym kawałku ciała Już nie mogę Was dłużej niszczyć Wybaczcie mi już nie mam siły walczyć choć tak bardzo chciałabym być z Wami.

Bardzo bardzo Was kocham ale Wy musicie żyć dalej.

**Extract 8**

Nie mogę wytrzymać szumu w uszach i tych tabletek.

Mama.

Ja i tak byłam nie do życia.

**Extract 9**

Córuchny kochane zawsze przy Was będę. Kocham was i nie smućcie się już będę wolny. [...] i kochane moje ja Was bardzo kocham ale już nie mam sił zawsze duchem będę przy Was.

**Extract 10**

[first name] wybacz mi, że Cię zawiodłam ale widzę, że gaśniesz, im dłużej tu będę tym bardziej Cię zniszczę a Ty musisz żyć dla dzieci.

Ja nie mam żadnych szans fizycznych. Bardzo Was kocham i będę kochała.

**Extract 11**

Bardzo Was kocham i będę kochała w każdej chwili nawet wtedy kiedy mnie już nie będzie. Wybaczcie mi że zabrałam Wam radość i młodość, że zadałam Wam tyle przykrości.

**Extract, 12**

Przepraszam że nie będzie mnie przy Twojej pierwszej komunii przy pójściu do szkoły i że nie będę mógł patrzeć jak dorastasz. Chcę żebyś wiedział że kocham Cię bardzo mocno i część mnie zawsze będzie przy Tobie.

**Extract 13**

Wasza trójka to jedyna, największa miłość mojego życia. Byliście moimi najcenniejszymi skarbami. Zawsze będę przy Was, zawsze będziecie czuć moją obecność. Wiem, że będziecie szczęśliwe.

**Extract 14**

Najukochańsze dzieci Syn [first name] i [first name] dbajcie o siebie [first name] i [first name] też. Najdroższe moje wnuki – [first name], [first name] [first name] i [first name] jestem z Was b. dumna że jesteście tacy wspaniali nie żalicie się i dbajcie o siebie w przyszłości o zdrowie i miłość. Chodźcie do kościółka i módlcie się

**Extract 15**

Kocham Cię i najtrudniej mi odejść bo nie mogę Cię nawet na koniec zobaczyć dwa dni patrzyłem na Twoje zdjęcie i płakałem ze szczęścia że mam tak cudownego syna.

Twój zawsze kochający Cię tata.

**Extract 16**

Dbaj o mamusię i bądź grzeczny i przede wszystkim nie słuchaj babci [first name] bo jest tępa i tylko potrafi niszczyć ludzi ucz się pilnie i rób to co czujesz i dąż do celów. Jesteś cudownym facetem i wszystko jest dla Ciebie możliwe.

**Extract 17**

[first name], [first name] i [first name] – kocham Was.

**Extract 18**

synu mój kochany, nie gniewaj się, że odchodzę – kocham Cię

Twoja matka

**Extract 19**

DZIECIAKI MOJE

[person_name] KOCHAM WAS

**Extract 20**

Kochałem tylko Ciebie.

**Extract 21**

[first name] KOCHAM CIĘ NAD ŻYCIE

ODCHODZĘ PRZEZ TWOJĄ MAMĘ

[first name] BARDZO CIĘ KOCHAM

**Extract 22**

[person_name] wiem że mnie nienawidzicie, ale chcę abyście wiedzieli że postąpiłam w ten a nie inny sposób, bo moje nerwy nie wytrzymały.

**Extract 23**

Jeszcze jedno mam nadzieję że teraz jesteście zadowoleni, wreszcie nie będziecie mnie wyganiać z domu.

**Extract 24**

[first name]. – Widziałem cię na cmentarzu – ale do mnie nie podeszłaś. – chyba mnie się wstydziłaś.

Ojciec.

**Extract 25**

Mimo to ze mnie nie za bardzo lubisz ale wiem kto cię do tego namawia. Nie bądź taka pyskata jak mama bo będzie Ci w życiu bardzo źle. Przecież byłaś za mną a nagle trach, już nauczyła włóczyć Cię po sądach i policjach. Życzę Ci abyś całe życie była zdrowa, ukończyła wszystkie szkoły które sobie wybierzesz oraz jak będziesz wychodziła za mąż to się dobrze zastanów. Ja już Ci błogosławię..

**Extract 26**

won i z chaty kurwo ty mnie ty niepotrzebna suko ty tichałaś i jebałaś zabieraj wszystko swoje i wypierdalaj

**Extract 27**

[First name] Ty dobrze wiesz dlaczego ja to zrobiłem, a jeśli masz wątpliwości to zapytaj mamusi; ja jestem tylko Waszym ojcem i bardzo Was kochałem, ale mama zniszczyła mi życie, chciała żyć bogato dostatnio i to jej się udało, zawsze marzyła o bogatym życiu, lecz Ty jako moja córka będziesz mnie miała do końca życia na sumieniu, i nie myślcie sobie że już byłem tak głupi, że mama zrobiła mi wycieczkę do USA ja wszystko zrozumiałem, dzieci które kochałem bardzo mocno zdradziły mnie.

**Extract 28**

Pamiętajcie też, że macie nienawidzić Waszego ojca [first name] [last_ name], bo on nie miał szacunku dla mnie i nigdy nie będzie miał go dla Was.

# 7 Legacy of the Self

## Introduction

In the previous chapter, we explored discursive constructions of relationships in suicide notes written by parents and explicitly addressed to their children. We focused on how the writing parent portrayed their relationship with their child. We found three dominant patterns in the dataset. First, the position taken by the parent is predominantly one of experiencing the world; in the letters, the parents constructed themselves as thinking or feeling rather than doing. Second, the children were described in positive terms. Third, the children were explicitly positioned in a relationship with the writing parent and hurt the parent.

In this chapter, we continue to focus on stories of parents who took their lives. As we explore stories of the aftermath of parental suicide, we are particularly interested in what could be seen as the parent's legacy, and the impact of the deceased parent on the surviving child and their life.

### *Aftermath of Parental Suicide*

Parental suicide is one of the most distressing and traumatic events for a child. It has a profound life-changing impact, resulting in the permanent loss of their children's critical attachments (Luecken & Roubinov, 2012). Parental suicide is particularly disruptive when it occurs during childhood or adolescence, a time when parents are the primary source of love, security and stability (Andriessen et al., 2020; Feigelman et al., 2017). It usually disrupts family balance and separates children from their peers (Andriessen et al., 2020; Carter & Brooks, 1991).

Studies have examined the effects of parental suicide on the children's physical, social, and psychological well-being. Researchers focused on the psychological consequences of parental suicide, including comparing outcomes in those bereaved by parental suicide with other causes of

DOI: 10.4324/9781032672847-7

parental death (Pfeffer et al., 2000; Brown et al., 2007). The discussion on the relationship between bereavement after suicide and death for other reasons is still ongoing; however, several research papers suggest similarities with grief themes, grief processes, and grief outcomes (Andriessen et al, 2017; Jordan, 2020; Sveen & Walby, 2008).

Researchers have also identified an increased risk of mental health complications (Andriessen et al., 2017; Brent et al., 2009) and suicidal behaviour in children who lose a parent to suicide (Calderaro et al., 2022), or other external causes compared to those who die naturally (Andriessen, 2020). Parental suicide is associated with an almost threefold increased risk of death by suicide and an almost twofold increased risk of attempted suicide, compared with children living with both parents (Caladeraro et al., 2022). The increased vulnerability can be attributed to a complex interplay of psychological, environmental, and social factors that act in conjunction with one another following the sudden death. Some of these include the child's age (Garssen et al., 2011; Niederkrotenthaler et al., 2012), gender (Hart et al., 2022; Cheng et al., 2014; Kaplow et al., 2010), the gender of the deceased parent (Goodday et al., 2019; Kuramoto et al., 2010), the child's mental health (Haine, Ayers, Sandler & Wolchik, 2008), the surviving parent's behaviour (Hung & Rabin, 2009), and the broader environmental support (Caladerado et al., 2022; Ratnarajah & Schofield, 2007; Pitman et al., 2016; Schreiber, Sands, & Jordan, 2017). For example, children who lost a parent or a primary caregiver at a relatively young age—particularly those under the age of six—are at greatest risk of developing long-term mental health issues, including suicidal ideation and attempts (Carpio et al., 2021). Typically, children who lost a parent to suicide experience changes in the quality of parenting from the surviving grieving parents (Calderaro et al., 2022); thus, children from families characterised by poor communication and high levels of conflict are more vulnerable to mental health problems following parental suicide (Hart et al., 2022).

Another factor that may affect the bereaved child is a suicide note left by the parent. However, research on parental suicide notes is scarce. Feigelman and co-authors (2019) found that there were no significant differences in the mental health outcomes of bereaved individuals who received a suicide note (mainly first-degree relatives) and those who did not (Feigelman et al., 2019). Researchers also found that individuals who expected to be suicidal but were not had more grieving difficulties and worse mental health (Feigelman et al., 2019).

Feigelman's research looks at a broad group of suicide survivors, while Giles analysed letters written by parents to their children (Giles, 2007). Giles' study shows that parents were more likely to leave notes (47%) than non-parents (33%). There were no significant gender or age differences, with more than 45% of both male and female parents and 40% of parents in all age groups (young, middle-aged, and older adults) writing notes (Giles, 2007). Giles also noted that letters to children often resembled gift messages. In this case, they typically focused on positive affirmations about the recipient and offered advice, albeit without providing practical instructions or explanations for the suicide. Giles argues parents continued to fulfil their roles and responsibilities, whether in partnership or as parents through these letters. Another study we found on parental notes was Utriainen and Honkasalo's (1996) semiotic analysis of suicide notes written by Finnish women. They showed that the content of notes addressed to men differs from that of notes addressed to children. They further argued that children received fewer conflicting notes, and they were full of the mother's love and longing (Utriainen & Honkasalo, 1996).

Although parental suicide is discussed in the literature, there is a paucity of research on suicide notes written by mothers and fathers to their children. Those suicide notes are usually the last messages from parents, and they can play an important role in the bereavement process and children's future relationship with the deceased parent. Therefore, in this chapter, we focus on messages about the future in parental suicide notes.

We focus only on suicide letters in this chapter. Suicide letters offer us insight into the messages sent in the context of the approaching suicide. We did not want to approach the ex-post-facto perspective mediated by the concerns of the moment of the interview. Moreover, for ethical reasons, we did not have access to the information about the marital or parenthood status of our interviewees. This is why consistent questioning about the parent's perspective was not possible. At the same time, our interviewees did not volunteer stories about the thoughts of their children at the time preceding suicide action.

## The Grand Legacy

In this section, we discuss suicide letters whose message was to offer the surviving child or children a gift after the parent's suicidal death. Two kinds of gifts were offered. On the one hand, there were messages bequeathing something with pecuniary value. Such gifts were explicitly positioned as gifts. On the other, the parental legacy was more ambivalent. Such legacies were symbolic and consisted of advice or care.

Consider the first four extracts in which the gifts resulting from suicide are described in explicit, direct terms:

### Extract 1

I leave you [amount in cash]. There is some money in institutions [social security].

**Extract 2**

> Take the grass mower, there is a cord broken there, but I bought it so ask your uncle [first name] and he will fix it for you. I wanted to buy a motorbike for you but because of your mum I ran out of money, it was taken by the courts and other institutions.

**Extract 3**

> You will have money because you will have benefits after my death. [...] you will be getting it as long you study.

**Extract 4**

> Please forgive me but I am doing it so that you will have a benefit after my death.

The first two extracts position the gift directly. In Extract 1, the author bequeaths an amount approximately equivalent to a minimum monthly wage at the time in Poland. In Extract 2, a gardening device is given. In both cases, the notes explicitly pass the money or the device to the addressees. However, Extracts 3 and 4 are different; the gift is contingent upon the death of the parent. In Extract 3, suicide seems written into legal regulations that stipulate that underage children, or those in full-time education, receive social benefits following their parent's death. In contrast, the author of the note in Extract 4 makes a direct link between his suicide and the money that will result from his suicidal death. His suicide is positioned explicitly as a means of financial gain for the children.

Now, what is crucial in these notes is that they were written by men, the fathers of the addressees of the notes. We suggest that such notes are anchored in the dominant views of fatherhood. The father's 'success' is measured by his interaction with the child, but also, crucially, by how he interacts with society (Zoja, 2001). Indeed, Zoja adds that children themselves want the father to succeed in the world; they want him to be strong and victorious.

This is the imagery and expectation of what Burgess (1997) calls the archetypal father: the king, the father in heaven, and a figure that is imbued with authority and power. The ever stronger pressure to provide is firmly coupled with women's claims to the traditionally masculine spheres of life (Featherstone, 2009; Miller, 2011). Such expectations are complicated by the changing fatherhood metanarratives. Fathers' absences from families are coupled with pressure for 'new fatherhood' and emotional involvement with the child (Dermott, 2008; O'Brien, 2005).

In the notes we quoted above, the father's suicide, we propose, is the ultimate evidence both for caring and for providing. The father constructs himself as giving his life for the children's financial security. It is the grand legacy of the father for their child, constructed by the ultimate sacrifice. It must be added, however, that there is only a handful of such notes written from the subject position of the father (there were significantly more notes in which the suicide author either did not identify himself or identified, for example, as a husband).

We would like to finish this section with two extracts offering some more nuance to the discussion above. Consider first the following letter:

**Extract 5**

> You will be on your own, with [first name], without us. Mum did not want to experience pain and suffering, and I did not see continuing life without her. We loved you very much and helped every way we could. Perhaps you will understand what life is like and perhaps the benefit you will get after our death will help you bounce back and stand on your own feet. Do not be embarrassed to seek advice from [first names] because they will now be your closest family.

In this letter, while suicide leads to a desirable outcome, it is not explicitly positioned as intended to bring the outcome about. The money the addressee is entitled to receive is a side effect of the suicidal act. Suicide is not positioned as a gift or even leading to a gift. Rather, it is positioned as a context for reflection about one's life.

Yet, just as in the extracts at the beginning of the chapter, suicide is represented as leading to something good, an outcome to be seen in positive terms. Significantly, it is the reflection on what life is like that is represented as linked to the child's being on her own and, in the process, leading to more understanding. The money is outside these considerations. The legacy of the parents taking their lives is offering their daughter space to reflect on herself.

Consider now the final extract of the section:

**Extract 6**

> Take care of your dad, I love him so much and I cannot torment him anymore. He has aged a lot, take care of him as much as you can.

Even though the author of the letter explicitly addresses her children, the suicide gift is not for them. What is significant in this letter is that the children are co-opted into taking care of their father following the mother's suicide. The children are asked to pick up the pieces after their mother's suicide; the mother's legacy might well be quite unwanted.

In this section, we discussed suicide as the ultimate legacy for the children. Suicide is portrayed as leading to good and desirable outcomes. In the extreme, suicide is committed for the outcomes to be brought about.

### Little Legacies

The grand legacy cannot be matched by other gestures of care or symbolic gifts. Yet, both fathers and mothers express their care in their letters. There are two ways in which this is done. First, parents' suicide notes contain what can be seen as life advice. Second, they also contain expressions of love and care.

Consider the following extracts:

#### Extract 7

Don't despair, try to live and bring [first name] up the way we brought you up. Have good memories of us and once in a while light a candle for us. Reflect on that we have always wanted best for you and your child.

#### Extract 8

You are the eldest. You will now be the host, and I know you will manage. Help your mum and take care of [first name] so no one hurts her. [first names], study because I had the opportunity but didn't take it.

#### Extract 9

Take care of yourselves, of your health and love. Go to church and pray. God is above us all.

#### Extract 10

I ask you for one thing very much. Love each other, respect each other and be together forever. You have only each other. But that' s much, very much.

All four extracts contain advice about how to be a 'good person' or how to lead a good life. This is advice that can stereotypically be seen as given by a parent, someone with greater experience, or someone in a position of some authority and with some cultural capital (Bourdieu, 1991).

The advice is underscored by the linguistic form. All the letters are written with the use of verbs in the imperative mood. This makes them more akin to orders or commands; as such, they can only be given by an elder. In this way, the letters are the final construction of parenthood and are the final words of wisdom for the children.

The letters also contain more concrete advice. Extracts 7 and 8 advise the addressees to manage another child's upbringing. Interestingly, Extract 8 positions the parent's experience as good reason to take the advice. Interestingly, the parent's last words position him in not so good a light. However, this can be done in a much stronger way:

**Extract 11**

> Go to work, become a respectable person.[1] Because of my stupidity, I have fallen and haven't been able to manage. Ditch this stupid company you keep or you will go to the dogs.

The life advice is supported by the reference to the writer's stupidity and continues with a shift to more concrete advice about the addressee's friends.

The legacy proposed in the letters was not always positive. We would like to end with two extracts exemplifying this point. Consider:

**Extract 12**

> Dear [little] son, I hope that when you grow you, you understand certain matters and you will forgive me. I am sorry I will not be by your side at your first communion, when you go to school that I will not be able to see you grow up.

The letter positions the writing father as doing something (unsaid) that can be evaluated negatively and is something that needs to be forgiven. Interestingly, the forgiveness does not extend to the father's absence at the child's life milestones. The letter also assumes that when the child grows up, the father will still be of relevance in the child's life. He will be a presence that will have to be dealt with. The author-father leaves the child with a plea for forgiveness that comes from understanding in the future, hoping the understanding will offer some resolution. Significantly, the letter does not suggest that the resolution is for the child; rather, the resolution seems to apply more to the father.

The last extract we want to discuss is the following:

**Extract 13**

> Also, remember that you are to hate your father [full name] because he has never had any respect for me and will never have it for you.

This is the only letter from a parent in our dataset that urges the children to hate the other parent. As in the extracts above, the letter is an instruction. The phrase is direct and strong. The author uses the phrase *mieć + infinitive* (roughly an equivalent to 'be + infinitive' in English) instead of the more common imperative mood. Such a phrase leaves no room for interpretation as to its intent; it can only be intended as an order or instruction.

Significantly, the order of hatred is supported by an explanation which is not only related to the author of the letter but also to the addressees. This is presumably why the reference to the future is also conveyed with an unmodalised clause suggesting no doubt.

In this section, we examined the last words of advice for the children of their parents' suicide letters. Such letters serve two functions in our view. First, they offer life advice and the last words of wisdom for the children, intended for a better life for the addressees. Second, they are also messages that are constructed to come from the parent. Parenthood is not only constructed through explicit references to the identity of the writer. It is also done through the linguistic form suggesting that the speaker is a person of authority and experience.

### *Messages of Care*

In this section, we discuss expressions of care in the notes. Life advice in suicide letters that we discussed in the previous section is also accompanied by expressions of good wishes and parental care. Consider the following extract:

**Extract 14**

> Despite that you do not like me much, but I know who is urging you [to be like that]. Do not be so gobby as your mum because you will have it hard in life. After all, you were fond of me but suddenly, bosh, she has taught you to go round the courts and the police. I wish you to be healthy your entire life, to finish all school you will choose. And when you get married consider it well. I give you my blessing right now.

There is an interesting opposition created by the two foci of the letter—the references to the author's daughter and then to himself. The author negotiates the story of his daughter's attitude, seemingly attempting to avoid blaming her for it. While he starts with the statement of the daughter disliking him, the statement is mitigated by 'not much' and creating an external source of the disliking. This is underscored by the statement introduced *przecież*, rendered here with 'after all', which refers to the first statement in the note. It is a challenge to the daughter's dislike claimed in the first statement. At the same time, there is a contrast with the claim about going around police stations. Significantly, the source of the daughter's actions relating to police or courts is again positioned as instigated by her mother, absolving the daughter from full responsibility for the actions.

The nuanced avoidance of blame is supported by a shift in the story. As if ignoring what was said, the letter author offers his unqualified good wishes. The good wishes are supported by the blessing for the daughter's future marriage. This support and care for the daughter, we propose, is the primary function of the letter. The father's last words to his child are those of care and love, despite the daughter's attitude (indeed, note the 'despite' at the beginning of the extract). The note leaves the child with an image of a caring father who does not pay attention to the daughter's transgressions and one whose absence will be felt in the future. Now, consider:

**Extract 15**

My dearest, I love you very much, but I cannot manage any more. I will always be with you in spirit. Forgive [addressing many] me.

**Extract 16**

My dear beloved daughters, I will always be with you. I love you and do not be sad. I will be free now.

**Extract 17**

I love you and it is hardest to depart because I cannot see you even at the end. I have looked at your photograph for two days and I have been crying of happiness that I have such a wonderful son. Yours always loving you dad.

What is perhaps the most interesting aspect of the extracts above is that what remains after the parent's death is the parent. In Extracts 15 and 16, the presence is conveyed by clauses without qualifications—linguistically, they are as certain predictions as can be—but are augmented by the adverb 'always'. Significantly, the assurances of continuing presence are preceded by expressions of love. The love, it seems, will continue even after suicide.

Extract 17, in contrast, is more ambivalent. The reference to the father's presence coming again after confessions of love is stressed by the signature in which the father is described as always loving. There is also an internal contrast between the signature and the earlier reference to the father's departure, perhaps.

The expressions of love and the claimed presence, we argue, offer a counterbalance to suicide, the ultimate departure, which could presumably be seen as an utter lack of care. In the letters, the authors position themselves not only as parents but also as caring parents, undermining the social perception of suicide (see Kollareth et al., 2019).

Consider the next group of extracts in which the writing parents show their care through the positivity of encouragement and support.

**Extract 18**

You are young, you are entitled to life and happiness. Your life is in front of you. Many bad and good moments await you. I am not afraid for you. You are clever and will manage. I could not.

**Extract 19**

Do not be sad. I believe the sun will bring your good spirits and will to live back. Support each other.

**Extract 20**

My darling daughter, I did not want to hurt you. Love your children, they need you.

**Extract 21**

I love you very much, but you live on.

We would like to further the discussion of expressions of care with two extracts that show care but through delegation. Consider:

**Extract 22**

I apologise to everyone. Very much. [First name], be happy with [first name]. Let him take care of you. Get a trade, pass your A-levels.

**Extract 23**

[First name], take care of [first names] and do not let anything bad happen to them. You are the eldest, so this is why I am writing this. In bag, I have another letter.

The last words of the two mothers are to delegate the care for their children. We presume that such messages are also expressions of care, much like handing over the watch. The mothers' messages represent them as remembering about the safety or security of their children.

Just as we argued that fathers' suicide notes containing offers of financial gifts to their children were underpinned by the foundation of the dominant model of fatherhood, we suggest that the notes above (Extracts 22 and 23) are also made on the foundation of the stereotypical model of motherhood. If motherhood is founded on caring for children, the two mothers' notes attempt to extend their duties. Their messages are seemingly aimed at making sure that their children are taken care of. There will be someone who will take over the motherly duty of care.

We would like to end the chapter with one last group of extracts. These are messages with no legacy, with the parent's presence removed from the child's future.

**Extract 24**

I am sorry I have failed you so much. I am only asking you not to tell the children about their father.

**Extract 25**

Do not tell [first name] what happened because he is too little and may not understand it. He is the only person that kept me alive. And it is hardest to do because of him. I believe it will only be better for you.

**Extract 26**

Burn my photographs so the son will not have to see me. Why should he be ashamed of me? I could not make sure that his dad is with him and that he loves him. My heart is breaking at the thought that I will never see him again and I fear that he will not understand. I hope that when he grows a little, you [first name] will explain it all to him and you will tell him that it was hardest to leave this world because of him, because he is dearest of all dearest.

**Extract 27**

> You must be brave now because of the children. I think you will manage well without me, and I think you will be happy later. Raise them as you have so far, and they will grow up to be wonderful people. Please remember only the good moments. I apologise to you for the harm, I am really sorry. When they grow up, tell them they had a good father, but he was ill.

We quote these messages because they speak directly to the role of the parent in the future life of their children, although they are not addressed to the children themselves. In all four extracts, the writing men assume the position of a father only to make sure that they are, as fathers, silenced by the children's mothers. The request for silence (and silencing) is sometimes absolute (as in Extract 24 and perhaps in 25) or qualified as in the others.

The explanations the children might receive when they are older (Extracts 26 and 27) are anything but clear, apart from the reassurance of the father's love (Extract 26). In Extract 27, the request concerns maintaining the father's (sort of) positive image. It is worth adding that the writer's reference to his illness makes suicide more socially acceptable (Dahlen & Canetto, 2002).

The juxtaposition of a request to silence by the father with requests to reassure the children that their father had not been all that bad is significant. As we discussed throughout this chapter, parenthood, including fatherhood, is to be performed even after the parent's death, and the performance consists of some sort of care about the children's future.

## Conclusions

In this chapter, we discussed the aftermath of parental suicide. We were interested in the 'legacy' suicidal parents leave for their children. We discussed two kinds of legacies. On the one hand, there is a grand legacy—suicide is positioned as a path towards a desirable outcome. In some cases, suicide was committed to achieve certain outcomes. On the other hand, we discussed the little legacies. These were messages of advice—the last words of wisdom from the parent about to die. We also discussed the last messages of care. The parents about to die expressed continuing love and presence.

As we already observed, the analysed letters suggest the multifunctionality of the suicide note. They are not simply goodbyes, let alone expressions of feelings or suicidality. Instead, they serve multiple functions including bequests or support. Moreover, the linguistic form of the letters suggests that parental identities continue to be important in the suicide letters and, possibly, after the parent's death. Parenthood is not only constructed through explicit references to the identity of the writer. It is also done through the linguistic form, suggesting that the speaker is a person of authority and experience.

It is surprising, however, that parental identities can remain relevant to the parent throughout the suicidal process up to the time just before their suicidal death. The dominant models of fatherhood or motherhood continue to be referenced, at least for some parents who are about to take their lives. In other words, the regulatory frames provided by such models do not disappear in the face of death. Being a father or a mother seems to be as important after death as it is while alive. Although the research paradigm within which we operate does not allow us to make generalisable claims, we can say, however, that suicide does not have to stop parenthood.

The most significant point we would like to highlight concerning the two models of parenthood is that they seem to offer different spaces for suicide. As fathers are judged based on their success in life, which for the most part means financial success, the material legacy of a suicidal father is a direct link with the dominant stereotypes of fatherhood. Fathers seem to say, 'I leave but I leave you something to have', thereby concluding the fatherly duty.

Alternatively, the motherly duties are more difficult to fulfil in suicide. If the mother's primary stereotypical duties are caring for children, then suicide seems to go against such an expectation. One cannot care for their children and, at the same time, take one's life. Hence, mothers seem to be in a trap, which might, one could hypothesise, be protective.

Although we did not focus on mothers, our earlier research (Galasiński & Ziółkowska, 2013), suggests that suicide is constructed as considerably less available in women's narratives. For women, suicide is not only extremely negative but also something to be fought against. Suicide is beyond normal things. For men, on the other hand, suicide is represented more in terms of logistic execution, rather than agonising. Suicide solves a man's problem.

Furthermore, the centrality of motherhood in the lives of children, supported by local cultural narratives of motherhood, makes it impossible for a mother simply to disappear.

**Extract 28**

Dear [first name]. My [little] daughter

[…]

I know you will be ashamed a little because of me, but do not worry about it. You will forget, like I never existed.

Suicide notes such as Extract 28 above seem impossible for a mother, while available to a father. Fathers can vanish especially after leaving a gift, an inheritance. Also, it is significant that the writing father constructs his future absence as resulting from the child forgetting him. This, we think, is unspeakable in the context of a mother. Indeed, while fathers fairly frequently wrote about the silence surrounding them, we found no such letters from mothers.

However, some notes, both from mothers and fathers, attempted to 'square a circle' as parents promised unending love, and, in some cases, permanent presence. Such notes are often dramatic instances of attempts to bridge the gap between the biological reality of suicide and the social expectations of parents.

The next chapter is concerned with love in the stories of people who either took their lives or made a serious attempt to do so. We are primarily interested in how love is represented in the last farewells. However, we also want to analyse love in the narratives following a suicide attempt. Using the metaphor of the postcard, we also want to see how love is constructed in the full-length film, which Leenaars argues is essential to understanding suicide (Leenaars, 2004).

## Note

1 The phrase used in the original is *wyjść na ludzi*. It is an idiomatic phrase that means to turn out well as a person. It is often used in reference to someone who beat the odds and became a respectable person.

## References

Andriessen, K., Krysinska, K., & Grad, O. T. (2017). Current understandings of suicide bereavement. In K. Andriessen, K. Krysinska, & O. T. Grad (Eds.), *Postvention in action: The international handbook of suicide bereavement support* (pp. 3–16). Hogrefe.

Andriessen, K., Krysinska, K., Rickwood, D., & Pirkis, J. (2020). 'It Changes Your Orbit': The impact of suicide and traumatic death on adolescents as experienced by adolescents and parents. *International Journal of Environmental Research and Public Health*, *17*(24), 9356. https://doi.org/10.3390/ijerph17249356

Andriessen, K., Rahman, B., Draper, B., Dudley, M., & Mitchell, P. B. (2017). Prevalence of exposure to suicide: A meta-analysis of population-based studies. *Journal of Psychiatric Research*, *88*, 113–120. https://doi.org/10.1016/j.jpsychires.2017.01.017

Bourdieu, P. (1991). *Language and symbolic power*. Polity.

Brent, D., Melhem, N., Donohoe, M. B., & Walker, M. (2009). The incidence and course of depression in bereaved youth 21 months after the loss of a parent to suicide, accident, or sudden natural death. *The American Journal of Psychiatry*, *166*(7), 786–794. https://doi.org/10.1176/appi.ajp.2009.08081244

Brown, A. C., Sandler, I. N., Tein, J. Y., Liu, X., & Haine, R. A. (2007). Implications of parental suicide and violent death for promotion of resilience of parentally-bereaved children. *Death Studies*, *31*(4), 301–335. https://doi.org/10.1080/07481180601187092

Burgess, A. (1997). *Fatherhood reclaimed: The making of the modern father.* Vermilion.

Calderaro, M., Baethge, C., Bermpohl, F., Gutwinski, S., Schouler-Ocak, M., & Henssler, J. (2022). Offspring's risk for suicidal behaviour in relation to parental death by suicide: Systematic review and meta-analysis and a model for familial transmission of suicide. *The British Journal of Psychiatry*, *220*(3), 121–129. https://doi.org/10.1192/bjp.2021.158

Carpio, L. D., Paul, S., Paterson, A., & Rasmussen, S. (2021). A systematic review of controlled studies of suicidal and self-harming behaviours in adolescents following bereavement by suicide. *Plos One*, *16*(7), e0254203. https://doi.org/10.1371/journal.pone.0254203

Carter, B. F., & Brooks, A. (1991). Child and adolescent survivors of suicide. In A. A. Leenaars (Ed.), *Life span perspectives of suicide* (pp. 231–258). Springer. https://doi.org/10.1007/978-1-4899-0724-0_16

Cheng, C. C., Yen, W. J., Chang, W. T., Wu, K. C., Ko, M. C., & Li, C. Y. (2014). Risk of adolescent offspring's completed suicide increases with prior history of their same-sex parents' death by suicide. *Psychological Medicine*, *44*(9), 1845–1854. https://doi.org/10.1017/S0033291713002298

Dahlen, E. R., & Canetto, S. S. (2002). The role of gender and suicide precipitant in attitudes toward nonfatal suicidal behavior. *Death Studies*, *26*(2), 99–116. https://doi.org/10.1080/074811802753455235

Dermott, E. (2008). *Intimate fatherhood*. Routledge.

Featherstone, B. (2009). *Contemporary fathering: Theory, policy and practice.* Policy Press.

Feigelman, W., Rosen, Z., Joiner, T., Silva, C., & Mueller, A. S. (2017). Examining longer-term effects of parental death in adolescents and young adults: Evidence from the national longitudinal survey of adolescent to adult health. *Death Studies*, *41*(3), 133–143. https://doi.org/10.1080/07481187.2016.1226990

Feigelman, W., Sanford, R., & Cerel, J. (2019). Suicide notes: Assessing their impact on the bereaved. *Suicide & Life-threatening Behavior*, *49*(3), 859–867. https://doi.org/10.1111/sltb.12489

Galasiński, D., & Ziółkowska, J. (2013). Experience of suicidal thoughts: A discourse analytic study. *Communication & Medicine*, *10*(2), 117–127. https://doi.org/10.1558/cam.v10i2.117

Garssen, J., Deerenberg, I., Mackenbach, J. P., Kerkhof, A., & Kunst, A. E. (2011). Familial risk of early suicide: Variations by age and sex of children and parents. *Suicide & Life-threatening Behavior*, *41*(6), 585–593. https://doi.org/10.1111/j.1943-278X.2011.00050.x

Giles, S. P. (2007). *The final farewell: Using a narrative approach to explore suicide notes as ultra-social phenomenon.* (Unpublished Doctoral Dissertation). University of Liverpool, UK.

Goodday, S. M., Shuldiner, J., Bondy, S., & Rhodes, A. E. (2019). Exposure to parental psychopathology and offspring's risk of suicide-related thoughts and behaviours: A systematic review. *Epidemiology and Psychiatric Sciences*, *28*(2), 179–190. https://doi.org/10.1017/S2045796017000397

Haine, R. A., Ayers, T. S., Sandler, I. N., & Wolchik, S. A. (2008). Evidence-based practices for parentally bereaved children and their families. *Professional Psychology, Research and Practice*, *39*(2), 113–121. https://doi.org/10.1037/0735-7028.39.2.113

Hart, R. K., Christiansen, S. G., Reneflot, A., & Hauge, L. J. (2022). Adolescents' primary care consultations before and after parental suicide: Evidence from population-wide data. *European Child & Adolescent Psychiatry*, *32*(12), 2453–2462. https://doi.org/10.1007/s00787-022-02095-3

Hung, N. C., & Rabin, L. A. (2009). Comprehending childhood bereavement by parental suicide: A critical review of research on outcomes, grief processes, and interventions. *Death Studies*, *33*(9), 781–814. https://doi.org/10.1080/07481180903142357

Jordan, J. R. (2020). Lessons learned: Forty years of clinical work with suicide loss survivors. *Frontiers in Psychology*, *11*, 766. https://doi.org/10.3389/fpsyg.2020.00766

Kaplow, J. B., Saunders, J., Angold, A., & Costello, E. J. (2010). Psychiatric symptoms in bereaved versus nonbereaved youth and young adults: A longitudinal epidemiological study. *Journal of the American Academy of Child and Adolescent Psychiatry*, *49*(11), 1145–1154. https://doi.org/10.1016/j.jaac.2010.08.004

Kollareth, D., Allam, A., & Russell, J. A. (2019). On judging the immorality of someone having taken his or her own life. *Social Cognition*, *37*(6), 547–570. https://doi.org/10.1521/soco.2019.37.6.547

Kuramoto, S. J., Stuart, E. A., Runeson, B., Lichtenstein, P., Långström, N., & Wilcox, H. C. (2010). Maternal or paternal suicide and offspring's psychiatric and suicide-attempt hospitalization risk. *Pediatrics*, *126*(5), e1026–e1032. https://doi.org/10.1542/peds.2010-0974

Leenaars, A. A. (2004). *Psychotherapy with suicidal people*. Wiley.

Luecken, L. J., & Roubinov, D. S. (2012). Pathways to lifespan health following childhood parental death. *Social and Personality Psychology Compass*, *6*(3), 243–257. https://doi.org/10.1111/j.1751-9004.2011.00422.x

Miller, T. (2011). *Making sense of fatherhood: Gender, caring and work*. Cambridge University Press.

Niederkrotenthaler, T., Floderus, B., Alexanderson, K., Rasmussen, F., & Mittendorfer-Rutz, E. (2012). Exposure to parental mortality and markers of morbidity, and the risks of attempted and completed suicide in offspring: An analysis of sensitive life periods. *Journal of Epidemiology and Community Health*, *66*(3), 233–239. https://doi.org/10.1136/jech.2010.109595

O'Brien, M. (2005). *Shared caring: Bringing fathers into the frame*. EOC.

Pfeffer, C. R., Karus, D., Siegel, K., & Jiang, H. (2000). Child survivors of parental death from cancer or suicide: Depressive and behavioral outcomes. *Psycho-Oncology: Journal of the Psychological, Social and Behavioral Dimensions of Cancer*, *9*(1), 1–10. https://doi.org/10.1002/(SICI)1099-1611(200001/02)9:1<1::AID-PON430>3.0.CO;2-5

Pitman, A. L., Osborn, D. P., Rantell, K., & King, M. B. (2016). Bereavement by suicide as a risk factor for suicide attempt: A cross-sectional national UK-wide

study of 3432 young bereaved adults. *BMJ Open*, *6*(1), e009948. https://doi.org/10.1136/bmjopen-2015-009948
Ratnarajah, D., & Schofield, M. J. (2007). Parental suicide and its aftermath: A review. *Journal of Family Studies*, *13*(1), 78–93. https://doi.org/10.5172/jfs.327.13.1.78
Schreiber, J. K., Sands, D. C., & Jordan, J. R. (2017). The perceived experience of children bereaved by parental suicide. *OMEGA – Journal of Death and Dying*, *75*(2), 184–206. https://doi.org/10.1177/0030222815612297
Sveen, C. A., & Walby, F. A. (2008). Suicide survivors' mental health and grief reactions: A systematic review of controlled studies. *Suicide and Life-Threatening Behavior*, *38*(1), 13–29. https://doi.org/10.1521/suli.2008.38.1.13
Utriainen, T., & Honkasalo, M. L. (1996). Women writing their death and dying: Semiotic perspectives on women's suicide notes. *Semiotica*, *109*(3–4), 197–220. https://doi.org/10.1515/semi.1996.109.3-4.197
Zoja, L. (2001). *Father*. Brunner-Routledge.

## Appendix

### Extract 1

zostawiam wam sześćset czterdzieści złotych. urządzi ma trochę pieniędzy a reszta zlozu i zusu.

### Extract 2

Weź sobie tą kosiarkę linkową tam jest urwana linka to ją kupiłem wisi na kierownicy poproś wujka [first name] to ci założy. Miałem ochotę kupić ci simsonka, ale przez mamę brakło pieniędzy bo zjadły sądy i inne instytucje.

### Extract 3

Pieniądze będziesz miała bo rentę po mnie dostaniecie [...] dopóki będziesz się uczyć to będziesz dostawała.

### Extract 4

PROSZĘ CIĘ ABYŚ MI WYBACZYŁA, ALE ROBIĘ TO DLATEGO ABYŚCIE MIAŁY RENTĘ PO MNIE.

### Extract 5

Zostaniesz sama z [first name] bez nas, mama nie chciała przeżywać bólu i cierpienia, a ja nie widziałem dalszego życia bez niej. Kochaliśmy

Was bardzo i pomagali jak tylko mogliśmy, może zrozumiesz co to jest życie i może środki jakie dostaniesz po nas pomogą Ci się odbić i stanąć na nogi, a rady nie wstydź się zaczerpnąć od [first name], [first name], czy [first name] bo oni będą teraz tylko dla Ciebie najbliższą rodziną.

**Extract 6**

Dbajcie o Tatę, tak bardzo go kocham i nie mogę już dłużej go dręczyć bardzo się postarzał dbajcie o niego tak bardzo jak tylko potraficie.

**Extract 7**

Nie załamuj się, staraj się żyć i wychować [first name] tak jak my Cię wychowali miej dobre wspomnienie po nas i zapal nad grobem od czasu do czasu znicza i zadumaj że chcieliśmy zawsze dla Ciebie i dziecka dobrze.

**Extract 8**

Jesteś najstarszy i teraz ty będziesz gospodarzem a wiem, że dasz sobie radę. Pamagaj mamie i opiekuj się [first name] i żeby jej ktoś krzywdy nie zrobił. [first name] i [first name] uczcie się bo ja miałem możliwości ale nie wykorzystałem tego.

**Extract 9**

dbajcie o siebie w przyszłości o zdrowie i miłość. Chodźcie do kościółka i módlcie się. Bóg jest nad nami wszystkimi

**Extract 10**

Bardzo Was proszę o jedno. Kochajcie się, szanujcie i bądźcie zawsze razem. Macie tylko siebie. Ale to dużo, bardzo dużo.

**Extract 11**

Idź do pracy i wyjdź na ludzi. Ja przez swoją głupotę upadłam, nie dałam już rady. Rzuć to głupie towarzystwo bo zejdziesz na psy.

**Extract 12**

Kochany synku mam nadzieję że jak dorośniesz to zrozumiesz pewne sprawy i mi wybaczysz. Przepraszam że nie będzie mnie przy Twojej pierwszej komunii przy pójściu do szkoły i że nie będę mógł patrzeć jak dorastasz.

**Extract 13**

Pamiętajcie też, że macie nienawidzić Waszego ojca [first name] [last_name], bo on nie miał szacunku dla mnie i nigdy nie będzie miał go dla Was.

**Extract 14**

Mimo to ze mnie nie za bardzo lubisz ale wiem kto cię do tego namawia. Nie bądź taka pyskata jak mama bo będzie Ci w życiu bardzo źle. Przecież byłaś za mną a nagle trach, już nauczyła włóczyć Cię po sądach i policjach. Życzę Ci abyś całe życie była zdrowa, ukończyła wszystkie szkoły które sobie wybierzesz oraz jak będziesz wychodziła za mąż to się dobrze zastanów. Ja już Ci błogosławię..

**Extract 15**

kochane moje ja Was bardzo kocham ale już nie mam sił zawsze duchem będę przy Was.

Wybaczcie mi

**Extract 16**

Córuchny kochane zawsze przy Was będę. Kocham was i nie smućcie się już będę wolny.

**Extract 17**

Kocham Cię i najtrudniej mi odejść bo nie mogę Cię nawet na koniec zobaczyć dwa dni patrzyłem na Twoje zdjęcie i płakałem ze szczęścia że mam tak cudownego syna.

Twój zawsze kochający Cię tata

**Extract 18**

Jesteście młode, macie pełne prawo do życia i szczęścia. Wasze życie dopiero przed Wami. Czeka Was dużo złych i dobrych chwil. Nie boję się o Was. Jesteście mądre i dacie sobie radę. Ja nie umiałam.

**Extract 19**

Nie smućcie się. Wierzę, że słońce przywróci Wam pogodę ducha i siłę do życia. Wspierajcie się wzajemnie.

**Extract 20**

Moja córeczko kochana, nie chciałam Cię skrzywdzić – kochaj swoje dzieci one potrzebują Ciebie

**Extract 21**

Bardzo bardzo Was kocham ale Wy musicie żyć dalej.

**Extract 22**

Przepraszam wszystkich. bardzo: [first name], bądź szczęśliwa z [first name]. Niech się Tobą opiekuje. Zdobądź zawód, zdaj maturę.

**Extract 23**

[first name] zaopiekuj się [first name] i [first name] nie pozwól aby cos złego im się stało jesteś najstarsza więc dlatego Ci to piszę w torebce mam jeszcze jeden list.

**Extract 24**

Przykro mi, że Was tak bardzo zawiodłem. Proszę Cię tylko o to byś dzieciom nie mówiła o ojcu.

**Extract 25**

[first name] nie mów co się stało bo jest jeszcze za mały i może tego nie zrozumieć. Jest jedyną osobą która trzymała mnie przy życiu i najtrudniej mi to zrobić z jego powodu ale wierzę że będzie wam tylko lepiej.

**Extract 26**

Popal też moje zdjęcia coby syn nie musiał mnie oglądać po co ma się mnie wstydzić.

się do taty a przede wszystkim wziąć go na kolana i przytulić do siebie. Nie mogłem mu zapewnić że tata jest przy nim i że bardzo go kocha.

Serce mi się kraje na myśl że już go nigdy nie zobaczę i boję się że tego nie zrozumie. Mam nadzieję że jak podrośnie to mu wszystko [first name] wytłumaczysz i powiesz mu że najtrudniej mi było odejść z tego świata z jego powodu bo jest skarbem nad skarby.

**Extract 27**

Musisz teraz być dzielna ze względu na dzieci myślę że beze mnie dasz sobie radę myślę że później i tak, będziecie szczęśliwi. Wychowuj je jak dotychczas a wyrosną na wspaniałych ludzi. Proszę Cię pamiętaj tylko o tych dobrych chwilach przepraszam Cię za wszystkie krzywdy jest mi naprawdę przykro. Jak dorosną powiesz że miały dobrego ojca tylko był bardzo chory.

**Extract 28**

Kochana [first name]. moja córeczko.

[...]

Wiem że trochę będzie Ci wstyd za mnie ale tym się nie przejmuj, szybko zapomnisz jakbym nigdy nie istniał.

# 8 The Emotional Self

## Introduction

In the previous chapter, we focused on stories of parents who took their lives. We were interested in the stories of the aftermath of parental suicide. The goal was to examine the parent's legacy and the impact the deceased parent wants to have on the surviving child's life.

In this chapter, the last of our empirical explorations, we are interested in the love stories of people who either took their lives or made a serious attempt to do so. In 1973, Shneidman (1973) compared suicide notes to postcards and wrote:

> Suicide notes are often like a parody of the postcards sent home from the Grand Canyon, the catacombs, or the pyramids—essentially unimaginative, pro forma, and not at all reflecting the grandeur of the scene being described, or the grandeur of the human emotions that one might expect to be engendered by the situation.
>
> (Shneidman, 1973, p. 384)

Interestingly, like in the postcard, the most common motif in suicide notes is love.

This chapter aims to explore discursive constructions of love in suicide notes. We are interested in how love is represented in the last farewells. However, we also want to analyse love in the narratives following a suicide attempt. Using the metaphor of the postcard, we also want to see how love is constructed in the full-length film.

### *Love in Suicidology*

It is now widely accepted that mental health problems are the main reason for suicide (Pridmore, 2011; Marsh, 2010). The suicidal person is usually portrayed as mentally distressed and commits suicide while in a poor

DOI: 10.4324/9781032672847-8

mental state. Psychiatric publications lead the way, often taking the relationship between suicide and mental disorder for granted. For example, Moscicki (1997) states that mental illness is a prerequisite for suicide. In the widely recognised book, *Night Falls Fast: Understanding Suicide,* Jamison (2000) noted that an extensive body of research across Europe, the United States, Australia, and Asia consistently showed that most individuals who take their lives have underlying psychopathology. Similar assertions were made by Harris and Barraclough (1997), who point out that, according to psychological autopsy studies, 90% of those who died by suicide attempt had one or more mental disorders at the time of suicide.

Recently, the psychiatric understanding of suicidal behaviour has been further reinforced. In the latest edition of the classification system of mental disorders published by the American Psychiatric Association [APA] (DSM 5 and DSM 5 TR) in 2013 and 2022, suicidal behaviour disorder and non-suicidal self-injury are included as conditions for further study (American Psychiatric Association [APA], 2013; 2022).

When the theme of love appears in the work of suicide researchers, it tends to be on suicide representations in media. Otherwise, love is mainly considered in the context of relationships. As relationships are among people's most important social interactions, their breakdown can cause psychological distress, including suicidal thoughts and behaviour. In most cases, research has found that people who are in long-term relationships such as marriage are less likely to attempt suicide than those who are divorced, separated, or who have never been married (Kazan et al., 2016). Divorced people appear to have the highest risk of suicide compared to other non-married groups (i.e., widowed and never married) and married people (Edwards et al., 2024; Stack & Scourfield, 2015). Heartbreak seems to be especially devastating. According to Edwards and colleagues (2024), the impact of divorce is more pronounced for women. The authors explain it by disproportionate losses in household income, increased risk of poverty, and a greater likelihood of single parenthood for women than men following divorce (Edwards et al., 2024).

Analyses of the relationship between marital status and suicidal behaviour do not address the quality of relationships, or love as an emotional state. They all show that those who reported high levels of unresolved conflict in their relationship had higher levels of suicidal ideation, hopelessness, and depression in comparison with people who tended to resolve issues with their partner amicably, or who reported no conflict (Till, Tran, & Niederkrotenthaler, 2017). In their recent qualitative study, Fallahi-Khoshknab and co-authors (2023) argue that emotional instability increases the likelihood of suicide attempts by creating feelings of shame, humiliation, burden, worthlessness, and insignificance.

Love, as an emotional state, has been extensively studied by suicidologists, mainly in the context of suicide notes. Researchers analysing suicide notes have developed various typologies (Galasiński, 2017), and love is a relatively common theme in suicide notes identified by researchers. For instance, Shneidman and Farberow (1957) categorised the content of notes into three categories: discomfort statements, relief statements, and neutral statements. Discomfort statements encompass motifs of guilt, blame, and tension, while relief statements include pleasant and warm feelings, as well as love. Neutral statements fall neither into the discomfort nor relief category. Similar findings were reported by Freuchen and Grøholt (2015); they discovered explanations for suicide, declarations of love, and instructions. Canetto and Lester (2002) also point to love and achievement. They argued that concerns about love in relationships may be a dominant component of suicide motivation. In a similar vein, Giles (2007), following McAdams (1993), points out that 'power', representing the need for agency and independence, and 'love', representing the desire for connection and dependence, are among the most fundamental motivations in human life. However, love has rarely been analysed in detail. One of the more detailed analyses was presented by Giles (2007), who showed that even those who have experienced significant suicidal stressors are socially oriented in their suicide notes, and the end of a romantic relationship becomes the central salient theme.

## Love and Suicide

Let us start with the following extract:

**Extract 1**

> I am trying to squeeze two words out of me: I love you. I have never loved anyone in such a way in my life and I will never do (ha, good one, I will never do). When I see you, I want to be alive. Or better: I wanted to be alive. I have never had such good conversations with anyone, and no one has understood me like you. Let us be honest: I am fucking crazy about you. I have thought about you incessantly, everything was about you. Even at night, I have dreamed about you (no erotic subtext please). The worst was when you went away home. I wanted to sleep all days so the time would fly faster, so that I could see you again. I know you have only liked me, like many others, fortunately, I have learnt to live with it.

The extract is one example of many in which authors of suicide notes express love. In Extract 1, the love confessed is portrayed as overwhelming, which is reinforced linguistically by the clauses in active voice, representing the writer as the loving actor. The author is also cautious to avoid blaming the addressee for his love. In the last sentence, he implies that his love is not the reason for his suicide. The expression of love in Extract 1 is therefore perhaps the last confession, a way to be remembered as the one who loved the most. It is in line with many letters in which love is expressed and not constructed as related to the suicidal act.

Yet, there were many other letters in which love is constructed as related to suicide. In this section, we want to discuss how love is expressed in suicide notes and linked to suicide. We are interested in how love, commonly assumed to be a positive emotion, is related to an act that is commonly thought of as negative. We also discuss the two contrasting ways in which love is constructed in suicide notes. First, love is constructed as undying; it survives suicide. Second, love is constructed as the reason for suicide—the letter authors tell their addressees about its destructive force.

### *Undying Love*

Consider the following extracts:

**Extract 2**

I will always love you

**Extract 3**

I love you. You will always be in my heart.

**Extract 4**

I love you. I will always love.

**Extract 5**

I will love [her] till the end of her life.

These fragments are simple. They promise eternal love as if suicide is not putting an end to the man's feelings (see Galasiński [2017] on non-finality of suicide). The authors' love will simply continue to exist. There is an interesting limit to the author's love in Extract 5, which we also discussed in Chapter 5. The love, it seems, will last until it is not needed.

Interestingly, it is not only romantic love that is undisturbed by suicide. Consider:

**Extract 6**

I will carry you in my [little] heart and, I hope, I will take care, with father, and watch over you.

**Extract 7**

I will remember you the way you are.

Both extracts position the authors as agents in carrying the addressee in their hearts and in remembering. We realise that, in such cases, as in all the extracts we quote above in this section, it is tempting to think that such suicide notes refer to a spiritual afterlife. We do not wish to make such claims as there is no evidence of this, either explicit or implicit. Rather, we think that such extracts are expressions of continuing bonds that are proposed by those who are about to die. Consider two more extracts of this kind:

**Extract 8**

I will miss you. I will not be able to live without you. You will never disappear from my heart. I will remember you all the time. Please apologise to everyone for what I have decided. But it is my decision, and I have considered it carefully. I will always love you.

**Extract 9**

You have a part of me at home and you must bring her up and one day tell her about me. I love you [plural] with all my heart, with all the strength I have left. Forgive. I will always be close by. I love you forever [first name].

Extract 8 is striking in juxtaposing suicide with the reference to an undying love. The references to love are reminiscent of someone breaking up a relationship, as are assurances of a person disappearing from one's heart. They suggest that the person continues to live, albeit apart from the loved one. The assurances are contrasted with a statement of having considered the decision. We think that the reference to the decision is for justifying the suicidal action. The continuing presence of the author of the letter is also mentioned in Extract 9. The note underscores the love that presumably also results in the request to bring up the daughter. The assurance of presence seems to be positioned as support for the mother, perhaps also as a suggestion that the author deserves to get the request granted and fulfilled.

Suicide is constructed as not ending the love, carrying in the heart, or remembering. Moreover, linguistically, such promises are made with clear references to the writers' agency in carrying them out, perhaps as a bid to reciprocate the love. There is a stereotypical way in which love is confessed. The repetitions of 'I love you' seem to almost imply eye contact between the lover and the loved one.

As we suggested in Chapter 5, such narratives are likely to be aimed at creating and maintaining a bond between the person who is about to take their life and the addressee. We also think that the narratives of unending love have an additional function. Love, we think, is assumed to be a symmetrical feeling; it should be reciprocated. The bond created by stories of love, therefore, goes beyond one that is created by the authors of the letters for the addresses. We suggest that such letters also impose a reciprocal bond; the addressees are at least implicitly asked to love the person back.

Indeed, such an argument is supported by the following extracts in which the confession of love is followed by a request for reciprocation.

**Extract 10**

I love you with my whole heart, you are my life. Never forget about this regardless of what happens.

**Extract 11**

I love you, do not ever forget about it. Think of me sometimes, and best once a month bring a white rose to my grave. I will know that you haven't forgotten me.

**Extract 12**

I love you, never forget the crazy man who loved you the most in the world. You are wonderful.

Such extracts reverse the perspective. Confessions of love are underscored by requests to remember it. The 'forever' or 'never' seem to raise the stakes for the addressees of the letters. Addressees are asked to continue the bonds that, as we suggest, are implied to be deserved because of the love offered. Love deserves reciprocation and, at the very least, must be acknowledged by remembrance. Furthermore, requests to remember are typically rendered in direct terms. There is no mitigation and there are no negative politeness (Brown & Levinson, 1987) strategies minimising the imposition. Instead, the requests are conveyed through clauses in the imperative mood, the default linguistic form in which to render directives.

Consider now one last extract in which the request goes even further:

**Extract 13**

> I apologise to you [plural] again, [first name]. Remember me the way I was. And love me for it. I love you very much.

The note is a request for reciprocating love. It is, once again, supported by the author's love and rendered in direct terms, with no qualifications. The bond requested by the author of the letter consists of an active emotional engagement from the addressee. Moreover, the love in question is not romantic. Although we have no access to the details of the relationships the author had with the addressees, the context would suggest that she is writing to her family or other close ones.

In this section, we have discussed constructions of undying love in suicide letters. There are two main arguments we made. First, the love referenced in the letters is well anchored in narratives of romantic love—all-conquering and ever lasting. However, also references to the non-romantic love tap into such stories. Second, we argued that the references to love surviving suicide have nothing to do with spirituality or an afterlife of sorts. Rather, we think that such notes' primary function is to set up an active reciprocal bond between the note writer and the addressee of the letter, which goes beyond their suicidal death.

### *Destructive Love*

In this section, we are interested in constructions of destructive love. The feelings of suicide letters' authors are positioned as contributing to their suicide. Love is represented as unwanted and, at the same time, unbearable. Still, the authors carefully manage responsibility for their love and suicide. In such notes, they often remove the object of their love from their accounts of suicide.

**Extract 14**

> You have been, you are, you will be the only person I have loved, I love, and I will love. You and [first name] are the sense of my life.

Unfortunately, we cannot be together, and I do not want to live without you. I am sorry you do not believe me, but, well, perhaps you will believe me now. Do not worry it is not yours, but it is my fault.

**Extract 15**

I hoped everything would work out between us, that you would love me as much as I have loved you.

**Extract 16**

I shall say one thing, it is because of my love for you. Farewell. Bye, bye.

The three extracts above can be seen on a spectrum of strength of the contribution of the thwarted love to suicide. Extract 14 sets up an opposition between the author's love and the addressee's inability to be with them, implying the addressee's lack of reciprocation. This contrasts with Extract 15, where the opposition lies in the unmatched love of the letter author for the addressee. Finally, Extract 16 explicitly positions love for the addressee as the reason for suicide. What is significant in those letters, however, is that they all can be seen to mitigate the blame apportioned to the addressees. The explicit reason for suicide in Extract 14 is the inability to be together—with no reference to the addressee's feelings. Extract 15 contains a reference to the hope of what could have been without any mention of the suicide causes. Extract 16, finally, only mentions the letter author's love and does not mention the addressee or her love.

Indeed, even a highly dramatic letter from a young woman stops short of an explicit accusation:

**Extract 17**

Now you have another proof what a girl in love and in despair is capable of doing when her beloved does not want her. I sacrifice it all, my parents, my siblings, [first names]. Generally, I am leaving my whole family in sadness and grief.

As in the previous letters, Extract 17 contains implications but stops short of an accusation. This is typical of the notes we found. The destructive love seems to be one-sided. The object of the love is not, at least in the linguistic form, implied in the suicidal action taken. Admittedly, we do not have a good explanation for such constructions, apart from a supposition that a straightforward accusation could be seen as undermining the love confession. Also, an accusation in a person's last words might be considered to be of special significance. In other words, the note writer does not want to leave the loved one with such a memory of them. Implication is enough.

Interestingly, even when the addressee is explicitly positioned as rejecting the author of the letter, they are not blamed for suicide.

**Extract 18**

Your goodbye put a damper on me even more. I do not know what made you do it. For seven months which I have been with you, I have loved you all the time.

**Extract 19**

The person I have loved has doubts in me, so I have doubts in myself.

The rejections in Extracts 18 and 19 are attributed to a concrete person. Yet, at the same time, the letters do not suggest blameworthiness. Things change, however, when the addressee of the letter is not the recipient of the author's love. Indeed, so far, we have discussed letters that were addressed to the loved one. In the letters where authors tell their story in the third person, the relationship between love and suicide changes into a much more direct one. Consider the following extracts:

**Extract 20**

Understand that I cannot manage like that anymore. I have been finished, removed from play. Is it a sin that I love him with all my heart? And he doesn't. And hates me on top of that.

**Extract 21**

I have decided to take my life for the reason that my wife [first name] married me, we had a child [first name] but she has never loved me and has hidden everything from me.

**Extract 22**

I apologise to you all for what I have done but I could not live like that knowing that my husband loves another woman and does not even notice his children.

**Extract 23**

She told me that I was to leave her alone that she wants me to disappear from her life. Without her life does not make sense for me. I love her and the only way to not to go to see her is to finish with myself. [...] I cannot see another solution in my life, without her, I cannot see any sense in living. I am certain that I wanted to spend my entire life with her. Without her, I can only see darkness.

References to killing oneself are explicitly related to the love felt towards a person. The four extracts above make the link in different ways. In Extract 20, the reference to the author's inability to continue living is linked to the beloved person not returning love. Extracts 21 and 22 contain references to the decision stemming from being not loved. Finally, Extract 23 is the most fulsome account of the author's inability to live.

It is significant, however, that love and lack of reciprocation are not positioned as the only reasons for taking one's life. Love does not seem to be enough and is placed next to hate, deception, and not being able to stay away. Indeed, when love is all that is spoken about, the message is softened, as in Extract 24. The source of suicide is rejection, but the well-wishing makes the message less aggressive and mean.

**Extract 24**

I loved her and I could not bear the thought that she rejected me.
I wish her happiness.

The negotiation of love as the source of suicide can be observed in the following extracts:

**Extract 25**

Tell [last name] that I have always loved him and will never forget him. Best show him this letter. I have fucked myself over because of him. He was the only boy I cared about. I wanted to kill myself for him. Which I have just shown. I loved being with him and he was just messing about. Tough. [first name], we shall never go to a disco together.

**Extract 26**

Hello everybody.
Ha, ha, I am not exactly laughing, are you? Do not fuss!
I am changing myself, but I get a kick from life. Fucking hell!

Forgive me…[speaking to many]
I love you all.
[first name]

In Extract 25, two moments in the letter suggest responsibility. The first one is the phrase 'zajebałam się', which we translated as 'I fucked myself over'. The Polish verb *jebać* is an all-purpose vulgarism, whose literal meaning is 'to have sex', or 'to fuck'. Here, it is used in its perfective aspect *zajebać*, which is normally used to refer to stealing, getting tired, and also killing. The phrase in the letter can be read as referring to suicide, yet the self-reference with such a verb strikes us, first-language users of Polish, as odd. The phrase might mean getting into trouble, getting confused, or getting forlorn in love. In the context, it is likely, we think, that the verb refers to suicide.

The second moment in the letter is the reference to wanting to commit suicide for the object of the author's love. There is another ambivalence here, however. The first statement is about killing herself 'for' the boy and not because of him, making the statement a proof of love instead of an ascription of blame. There is no way of knowing what exactly went through the author's mind. A close reading of the text suggests ambivalence that cannot be easily dispelled through language analysis.

In Extract 26, the author writes about 'a kick from life', which follows his change. Linguistically, the person for whom the author changed is not mentioned, and there is hardly any textual implication that the person is to be blamed for what was about to happen. However, even though there is no ascription of responsibility in the linguistic form, we think that, socially, such implications are likely to be received.

It is worth noting that our dataset includes suicide letters that express blame directly. These notes are presented below:

**Extract 27**

You killed. You killed. You killed. You killed.

**Extract 28**

You have got what you wanted.

**Extract 29**

Farewell, you will not torment and beat me. I give you a free hand.

Significantly, such notes do not contain confessions or promises of love. The notes invoke connotations of tragic, sorrowful love that results in death. Yet, love is never mentioned alongside casting blame. As we discussed earlier, it appears that confessing love while simultaneously blaming the recipient for causing suicide is socially unacceptable and would undermine the confession. Our analysis of suicide letters suggests that while an individual cannot, or perhaps should not, blame another for the absence of love, they can express blame for unbearable behaviour. While one cannot demand love, it seems, one can demand appropriate behaviour. Indeed, this can mean blaming oneself.

**Extract 30**

> I have been a bad wife and mother. I cannot live like that any longer.

We would like to conclude this section with one final extract in which love appears to end in such a way that it becomes the reason for suicide:

**Extract 31**

> You recently said that you would twist my head dead,[1] or you will tear them out with your bare hands. I would never have expected that of you because I considered you as everything that is the most beautiful and the most wonderful. But you showed your other face, calling me a monster. I listened to it and was silent because you are still this beloved [first name]. Still, despite all those words. Despite that, you hit me then in the car. I was very sorry, but I tried to explain it away every day. But I cannot anymore. I cannot and I do not want to. I want to die and shorten my pain and the suffering you caused me.

Extract 31 is a letter that lies between those expressing eternal love and those expressing destructive love. It is a story about a love that has been disappointed, yet it seems to endure. Interestingly, the story is primarily written in the first-person singular, focusing mostly on the author's experience. The author constructs the reason for her suicide as her inability to explain away what had happened. The pain caused by her partner comes only later and in the subordinate clauses.

We think the tension between the linguistic form and the social reading of suicide letters can be seen in most of the letters we quote. They are not merely expressions of love, damaging or not. We suggest that, socially, love is expected to be reciprocated. It is a gift, and gifts place the recipient under some obligation to reciprocate—in this case, to love back. The notes of damaging love, therefore, must not imply hurt from those to whom the love is confessed. In addition, destructive love is aimed at creating a lasting bond founded on negativity and, however subtly implied, blame.

In summary, we discussed love in suicide notes. There are two ways in which love is expressed. On the one hand, there is love that conquers all and endures beyond the suicidal act. On the other, love is portrayed as destructive and unwanted, both by the loving and the loved persons. We argued that both kinds of letters were intended to create a continuing bond with the addressees. The loving person will forever love and hence be present; the thwarting person will forever be in debt.

## Evidence for Love

In contrast to suicide letters, informants in the post-attempt interviews very rarely talked about love. In their stories, love was a proxy for relationships and their quality. In this section, we change the dataset we examine. We seek to explore the rare narratives of love in the accounts after a suicide attempt. Although references to love were rare, a clear pattern emerged from the data. Love consistently appeared only when the informants talked about their future (prompted by a question about how they see their future life) and was consistently positioned as protective.

In these narratives, love invariably comes from those close to the informant and is offered unconditionally. The informants position themselves as receiving the feelings, regardless of what transpired. Furthermore, the close ones' love is portrayed as providing the informant with a sense of purpose. Additionally, love was not only expressed but also supported by evidence.

Consider the following extract, which is part of an answer to a question about how the individual envisions her future:

### Extract 32

> I start thinking about my daughter. That now she made me realise that she showed me how much she loves me, how much she cares about me. And that my death would hurt her very much. Injure her. She said she didn't know whether she would cope. Whether she would come to terms with the situation and whether she would not make an attempt on her life herself. [...] It turned out that she loves me very much. She does not complain that I was not the best mother I could have been.

In the extract, love is constructed as a space in which there is no place for suicide. However, there are two other aspects of the story we want to explore. Both are concerned with how the daughter's declared love is evidenced and supported. First, the narrated love is given evidence in the form of the daughter's quoted words about her potential suicide. The informant repeatedly underscores that she quotes the daughter, presumably to attest to the veracity of the claims. Second, the story changes from quoting to a more 'objective' narrative when the informant introduces the verb *okazało się* ('it turned out'). The verb no longer reports on experiences or another's narratives; it introduces a reference to the extra-linguistic reality. The informant introduces factuality into her narrative. Such narratives are typical of the dataset. Consider also:

**Extract 33**

I have realised that my children do care about me. That I am really needed by them. That despite that they have their own families they do love me as a mother. Because they never told me that because they think it normal that I know that they love me. Because I am their mother, and they must love me.

**Extract 34**

The children showed me that I am, they said that I am still needed, that I have someone to live for because I have them and a husband. I have grandchildren whom I love greatly. But at that moment I was not thinking about anyone, only about myself, right?

**Extract 35**

The first days I spent being observed I was thinking why they had saved me. And later when my children started calling me, we started talking and writing to each other, thanks to my children I understood that I had made a big mistake because they really need me. It has like dawned on me that together with the children, that they are the most important. That I have hurt them.

The three extracts underscore the claims of love in different ways. In Extract 33, the informant uses 'really' to emphasise the claim, while, at the same time, she relies on the social practices of children's love for their mother. The children's perspective is also used in Extract 34, where the narrative starts with an appeal offered by the children. The claims are no longer only hers; they are introduced through argumentation. Such a rational foundation of the claims of love is also used in Extract 35, where the informant tells a story about communication and understanding, with the former resulting from a sort of epiphany.

Even though statements about love tend to be introduced by superordinate clauses, especially reported speech, they are all made without qualifications. The statements are in the present tense, implying their timelessness. Additionally, reported speech, especially coming from sources external to the informant, helps raise the credibility of the statements.

Moreover, verbs such as 'realise' or 'demonstrate' could be considered factive that is to say, they presuppose[2] the validity of the claim they introduce (Dahlman et al., 2022). In other words, a sentence such as 'I realised my children love me' presupposes that the children love the speaker. In the process, the claim about the children's love is assumed to be true, thereby strengthening its evidential basis. Consider:

**Extract 36**

> The children showed me that I am; they said that I am still needed, that I have someone to live for because I have them and a husband. I have grandchildren whom I love greatly. But at that moment I was not thinking about anyone, only about myself, right?

The initial 'show' that introduced the claim of being needed is put into a presupposition, and even though the verb 'say' is probably not factual, the veracity of the statement does not solely emanate from subjective experience.

In this section, we explored narratives about the love of the people close to those who had attempted to take their lives. There are two important patterns in the narratives. First, love is represented as preventing suicide. It creates a relationship in which suicide is too hurtful to commit. The second pattern is that love is consistently asserted not through experience, but rather with the aid of discursive devices that strengthen the claims and attests to their veracity.

Furthermore, the references to love create a relationship in which informants find a role. Being loved in such narratives means having a relationship whose source is in those who love. It opens space for the informant to fit into a life that is positive enough to be continued. In this way, love is not only protective but also creates relationships that are.

## Conclusion

In this chapter, we discussed love in relation to suicide. We started with how it is constructed in suicide letters. There are two ways in which love is expressed. On the one hand, there is love that conquers all and endures the suicidal act. On the other, love is destructive and unwanted, both by the loving and the loved persons. We argued that both kinds of letters are aimed at creating a bond between the writer and addressee. However, the undying love has the additional function of creating an active loving relationship with the addressee. Such letters appear to imply that love must be reciprocated.

When we focused on love narratives in post-attempt interviews, we found two patterns. First, love is represented as preventing suicide. Second, love is consistently claimed not through personal experience but with the help of discursive devices that make the claims more compelling and provide evidence of their truthfulness. Moreover, narratives of love make it transactional—it must be put into practice and reciprocated by both parties.

Now, in suicidology, love is studied predominantly in reference to media representations; we did not find any research on the relationship between love and suicide. Yet, our data show that love plays a significant role in suicide. In all the narratives, love is constructed as a dominant feeling. Whether it is all-encompassing undying love, or thwarted and destructive, it is constructed as having a significant position in the suicide process.

There are two points here to note. In our data, love is far from being a 'positive emotion' as it is often assumed to be in suicidological research (e.g., Barnes et al., 2007; Handelman & Lester, 2007; Pestian et al., 2010; Pestian et al., 2012). Love is complicated, and as much as it is constructed to be positive, it can also be unwanted. It also goes far beyond lexical references that are mostly studied in suicidology. We suggest that understanding love and attitudes towards it will significantly enhance our knowledge of suicide and its processes.

Our data analyses also show that the complex relationship between love and the suicidal process raises issues for suicide prevention and clinical work with the bereaved. For example, research still knows little about how assurances of love in suicide letters are received by letter addresses. Are such assurances welcome? Do they offer some succour? Alternatively, what is the reception of the notes telling stories of unwanted, destructive love? Our data suggest that such questions are important in understanding suicide, not only from the point of view of the person taking their life but from that of those who are left behind.

A commonly accepted view of suicide is understanding it in terms of emotionality, pain, and cognitive constriction. Several models of suicide focus on rejection, hopelessness, thwarted belongingness, and other implicit emotional responses to the world (e.g., van Orden et al., 2010; O'Connor, 2011). Galasiński (2017) argues that suicide notes do not support this view of suicide.

While certainly not consistently, love in suicide notes is constructed as far from the pain described by the dominant view. It may well be that such feelings are in parellel to other, more negative feelings, yet one must not see suicide only in terms of the 'negative' emotionality. Love is often constructed as the last words, possibly, as argued in the preceding chapter, the legacy of the suicidal person.

Let us consider the issue from a linguistic point of view. We need to briefly introduce the concept of modality. Modality is to do with the expression of the speaker's attitude towards the proposition they render in their utterance; the extent to which the speaker commits to, or distances themselves from what they say. The concepts that modality deals with are truth, and are related to necessity, possibility, as well as obligation and permission. Here, we are dealing with epistemic modality, the capacity of clauses to express the speaker's certainty as to what happened, or, their certainty that what they say is true. The certainty ranges from very low to very high (Halliday, 1994).

Notes referring to love are consistently at the highest level of certainty. Consistently, there are no qualifications or hesitations expressed in the them. The writers depict themselves as confident about the future. Love will happen, no matter what. The question of thwarted belongingness is challenged by such notes. Indeed, as the letters are read after their authors' deaths, the certainty of love or its presence could at least be seen as an attempt to communicate closeness and support, however non-physical it is. The promises and confessions are perhaps also assurances or consolations, with suicide almost brushed aside by the deceased person's love and its strength. As we suggested several times, some of the notes were reminiscent of representing a relationship breakup rather than death.

Suicide love letters also show how dilemmatic suicide is. We refer here to the notion of the ideological dilemma (Billig et al., 1988) and suggest that love in suicide letters appears to accomplish contradictory ideological stances between the suicidal departure and the loving presence. Suicide letters not only suggest the complexity of the love–suicide relationship but also the complexity of suicide itself.

Our interviews also offer valuable insights not only into the role of love but also into understanding the suicidal process. Love is narrated as having the power to allow those who tried to take their lives to see their future. However, the letters suggest that it is not simply love; it is a love that must meet certain conditions of reciprocity and must work. In the letters, the latter condition is constructed as being needed.

Furthermore, we argue that our interviews offer additional contexts to the issue of belongingness, which is central to suicide theory, though mostly referred to in negative terms. Both Joiner (2005) and later, van Orden et al. (2010), talk about thwarted belongingness without giving much thought to what exactly that belongingness is. Similarly, connectedness, another concept frequently used in understanding suicide, tends to be studied in terms of types of relationships. However, the Interpersonal Needs Questionnaire does not explore the 'content' of connectedness or belonging. One of the questions asks whether one belongs (*I feel I belong*) without exploring what it might mean.

In contrast, our data suggest that there is 'content' in such statements that can and should be explored. Stories of love in the interviews show the conditions necessary for love to count as protective. More importantly, the stories we collected show the importance of 'experiencing' love and having evidence for the feeling.

There are two aspects of such evidence. First, the evidence for love is constructed through the linguistic form of the narrative. Our informants' narratives focus on material or verbal processes, stressing the 'objectivity' of the claims of love. Second, such evidence also comes from the contents of the stories. Our informants focus on what their loved ones do, not only on how they are perceived. In addition, self-references, such as claims of being needed, are consistently made in relationship to the loved ones.

The data we presented in this chapter makes for two interrelated arguments. Not only is there no need to conceptualise belongingness in negative terms, but there is evidence that its positive representation is possible and needed. Furthermore, our interview data also suggested that belongingness is transactional.

This is the last empirical chapter of the book. In the next chapter, we present the main points of the book.

## Notes

1 The author of the note uses the phrase *ukręcić łeb,* which literally means 'to twist the head off'. The phrase is a linguistic cliché often used in jest. Our respective linguistic competences received the phrase as mildly unsettling, or at least, a serious threat, if not outright unusual.

2 Presupposition is a claim without whose truthfulness a sentence makes no sense. In other words, the implication carried by the sentence is necessarily true. For example, the sentence 'John has stopped writing' necessarily implies that John has written before.

## References

American Psychiatric Association [APA]. (2013). *Diagnostic and Statistical Manual of Mental Disorders (DSM-5).* American Psychiatric Publishing.

American Psychiatric Association [APA]. (2022). *Diagnostic and Statistical Manual of Mental Disorders, Fifth Edition, Text Revision (DSM-5-TR).* American Psychiatric Association Publishing.

Barnes, D. H., Lawal-Solarin, F. W., & Lester, D. (2007). Letters from a suicide. *Death Studies*, *31*(7), 671–678. https://doi.org/10.1080/07481180701405212

Billig, M., Condor, S., Edwards, D., Gane, M., Middleton, D., & Radley, A. R. (1988). *Ideological dilemmas*. Sage.

Brown, P., & Levinson, S. C. (1987). *Politeness: Some universals in language usage (vol. 4)*. Cambridge: Cambridge University Press.

Canetto, S. S., & Lester, D. (2002). Love and achievement motives in women's and men's suicide notes. *Journal of Psychology*, *136*(5), 573–576. https://doi.org/10.1080/00223980209605552

Dahlman, R. C., & van de Weijer, J. (2022). Cognitive factive verbs across languages. *Language Sciences*, *90*, 101458. https://doi.org/10.1016/j.langsci.2021.101458

Edwards, A. C., Ohlsson, H., Salvatore, J. E., Stephenson, M. E., Crump, C., Sundquist, J., Sundquist, K., & Kendler, K. S. (2024). Divorce and risk of suicide attempt: A Swedish national study. *Psychological Medicine*, *54*(8), 1620–1628. https://doi.org/10.1017/S0033291723003513

Fallahi-Khoshknab, M., Amirian, Z., Maddah, S. S. B., Khankeh, H. R., & Dalvandi, A. (2023). Instability of emotional relationships and suicide among youth: A qualitative study. *BMC Psychiatry*, *23*, 50. https://doi.org/10.1186/s12888-023-04534-0

Freuchen, A., & Grøholt, B. (2015). Characteristics of suicide notes of children and young adolescents: An examination of the notes from suicide victims 15 years and younger. *Clinical Child Psychology and Psychiatry*, *20*(2), 194–206. https://doi.org/10.1177/1359104513504312

Galasiński, D. (2017). *Discourses of men's suicide notes: A qualitative analysis*. Bloomsbury Publishing.

Giles, S. P. (2007). *The final farewell: Using a narrative approach to explore suicide notes as ultra-social phenomenon*. (Unpublished Doctoral Dissertation). University of Liverpool, UK.

Halliday, M. A. K. (1994). *An introduction to functional grammar* (2nd ed.). Edward Arnold.

Handelman, L. D., & Lester, D. (2007). The content of suicide notes from attempters and completers. *Crisis*, *28*(2), 102–104. https://doi.org/10.1027/0227-5910.28.2.102

Harris, E. C., & Barraclough, B. (1997). Suicide as an outcome for mental disorders. A meta-analysis. *British Journal of Psychiatry: The Journal of Mental Science*, *170*, 205–228. https://doi.org/10.1192/bjp.170.3.205

Jamison, K. R. (2000). *Night falls fast: Understanding suicide*. Vintage.

Joiner Jr., T. E. (2005). *Why people die by suicide*. Harvard University Press.

Kazan, D., Calear, A. L., & Batterham, P. J. (2016). The impact of intimate partner relationships on suicidal thoughts and behaviours: A systematic review. *Journal of Affective Disorders*, *190*, 585–598. https://doi.org/10.1016/j.jad.2015.11.003

Marsh, I. (2010). *Suicide: Foucault, history and truth*. Cambridge University Press.

McAdams, D. P. (1993). *The stories we live by: Personal myths and the making of the self*. The Guilford Press.

Mościcki, E. K. (1997). Identification of suicide risk factors using epidemiologic studies. *Psychiatric Clinics of North America*, *20*(3), 499–517. https://doi.org/10.1016/s0193-953x(05)70327-0
O'Connor, R. (2011). Towards an integrated motivational–volitional model of suicidal behaviour. In R. O'Connor, S. Platt, & J. Gordon (Eds.), *International handbook of suicide prevention: Research, policy and practice* (pp. 181–198). John Wiley & Sons.
Pestian, J., Nasrallah, H., Matykiewicz, P., Bennett, A., & Leenaars, A. (2010). Suicide note classification using natural language processing: A content analysis. *Biomedical Informatics Insights*, *2010*(3), 19–28. https://doi.org/10.4137/bii.s4706
Pestian, J. P., Matykiewicz, P., Linn-Gust, M., South, B., Uzuner, O., Wiebe, J., Cohen, K. B., Hurdle, J., & Brew, C. (2012). Sentiment analysis of suicide notes: A shared task. *Biomedical Informatics Insights*, 5(Suppl. 1), 3–16. https://doi.org/10.4137/bii.s9042
Pridmore, S. (2011). Medicalisation of suicide. *Malaysian Journal of Medical Sciences*, *18*(4), 78–83.
Shneidman, E. S. (1973). Suicide notes reconsidered. *Psychiatry*, *36*(4), 379–394.
Shneidman, E. S., & Farberow, N. L. (1957). Some comparisons between genuine and simulated suicide notes in terms of Mowrer's concepts of discomfort and relief. *Journal of General Psychology*, *56*(2), 251–256. https://doi.org/10.1080/00221309.1957.9920335
Stack, S., & Scourfield, J. (2015). Recency of divorce, depression, and suicide risk. *Journal of Family Issues*, *36*(6), 695–715. https://doi.org/10.1177/0192513X13494824
Till, B., Tran, U. S., & Niederkrotenthaler, T. (2017). Relationship satisfaction and risk factors for suicide. *Crisis*, *38*(1), 7–16. https://doi.org/10.1027/0227-5910/a000407
Van Orden, K. A., Witte, T. K., Cukrowicz, K. C., Braithwaite, S. R., Selby, E. A., & Joiner Jr. T. E. (2010). The interpersonal theory of suicide. *Psychological Review*, *117*(2), 575–600. https://doi.org/10.1037/a0018697

## Appendix

### Extract 1

Otóż próbuję z siebie wydusić dwa wyrazy: kocham Cię. Jeszcze nigdy w życiu tak nikogo nie kochałem i nigdy nie będę (he, dobre: nie będę). Kiedy Cię widzę to aż mi się chce żyć, a raczej chciało żyć. Z nikim innym nie rozmawiało mi się tak dobrze i nikt inny mnie nie rozumiał tak jak Ty. Bądźmy szczerzy: odjebało mi na Twoim punkcie. Bez przerwy tylko myślałem o Tobie, wszystko kojarzyło mi się z Tobą, nawet po nocach mi się śniłaś (tylko bez podtekstów erotycznych proszę). Najgorzej było, kiedy wyjeżdżałaś do domu. Chciałem wtedy spać całymi dniami żeby ten czas szybciej zleciał i żebym mógł Cię znowu zobaczyć.

Wiem, że Ty mnie tylko lubiłaś, jak wielu innych, na szczęście nauczyłem się z tym żyć.

**Extract 2**

Zawsze będę Cię kochał.

**Extract 3**

Kocham Cię i zawsze będziesz w moim sercu.

**Extract 4**

KOCHAM CIĘ ZAWSZE BĘDĘ KOCHAŁ.

**Extract 5**

[first name] będę kochał do końca jej życia

**Extract 6**

[first name] będę nosił Cię w serduszku i mam nadzieję że opiekował się z ojcem czuwał nad Tobą.

**Extract 7**

TAKĄ CIĘ ZAPAMIĘTAM.

**Extract 8**

Będzie mi Ciebie brakowało. Nie będę umiał żyć bez Ciebie. [...] Z mojego serca nigdy nie zginiesz. Przez cały czas będę o Tobie pamiętał. [...] Przeproś wszystkich że tak postanowiłem. Ale to jest moja decyzja i uważnie ją przemyślałem. Zawsze będę Cię kochał.

**Extract 9**

masz cząstkę mnie w domu musisz ją wychować musisz jej kiedyś o mnie powiedzieć kocham Was z całego serca ze wszystkich sił jakie mi pozostały wybacz zawsze będę blisko.

Kocham Cię na zawsze [first name]

**Extract 10**

Kocham Cię z całego serca jesteś moim życiem i nigdy o tym nie zapomnij bez względu na to co się stanie.

**Extract 11**

Kocham Cię i nigdy o tym nie zapomnij. Wspominaj mnie czasami, a najlepiej raz w miesiącu przynieś na mój grób białą różę będę wiedział że o mnie nie zapomniałaś.

**Extract 12**

Kocham Cię nie zapomnij o mnie nigdy, o tym wariacie który pokochał Cię najmocniej na świecie jesteś cudowna.

**Extract 13**

Przepraszam Was jeszcze raz [person_name] – „Pamiętajcie mnie taką jaką byłam"... i kochajcie mnie za to.

**Extract 14**

Byłaś, jesteś i będziesz jedyną osobą, kobietą którą kochałem, kocham i będę kochał ty i [first name] jesteście moim sensem życia niestety nie możemy być razem a ja bez was nie chcę żyć I szkoda że mi w to nie wierzysz ale cóż może teraz uwierzysz i nie martw się to nie twoja tylko moja wina.

**Extract 15**

Myślałem, miałem nadzieję że wszystko między nami się ułoży, że mnie pokochasz tak bardzo jak ja pokochałem Ciebie.

**Extract 16**

Powiem jedno to z miłości do Ciebie Żegnam Pa Pa

**Extract 17**

Teraz masz kolejny dowód na to co zakochana i zrozpaczona dziewczyna jest w stanie zrobić, gdy ukochany jej nie chce. Poświęcam wszystko Rodziców, rodzeństwo [first name], [first name], [first name], ogółem całą moją rodzinę zostawię w smutku i żalu.

**Extract 18**

To Twoje pożegnanie zgasiło mnie jeszcze bardziej. Nie wiem co skłoniło Cię do takiego ruchu

Przez siedem miesięcy które byłem z Tobą kochałem Cię cały czas.

**Extract 19**

Osoba którą pokochałam zwątpiła we mnie, więc ja zwątpiłam w siebie!

**Extract 20**

Ale zrozumcie, że już nie potrafię tak dalej, zostałam wykończona i usunięta z gry! Czy to grzech, że ja Go „KOCHAM CAŁYM SERCEM"?!!! A On mnie nie! i jeszcze nienawidzi!

**Extract 21**

postanowiłem odebrać sobie życie z tego powodu ponieważ moja żona [first name] wzięła ze mną ślub mieliśmy dziecko [first name] a ona nigdy mnie nie kochała ukrywała wszystko przede mną przede mną.

**Extract 22**

Przepraszam Was wszystkich za to co zrobiłam, ale dłużej nie potrafiłam już tak żyć wiedząc że mój mąż kocha inną kobietę i nie zauważa nawet własnych dzieci.

**Extract 23**

W każdym razie powiedziała że mam jej dać spokój i chce żebym zniknął z jej życia. Bez niej życie nie ma dla mnie sensu Kocham ją a jedyny sposób żeby do niej nie jeździć to ze sobą skończyć. [...] Innego wyjścia w swoim życiu nie widziałem bez niej nie widzę sensu życia.

Teraz jestem pewien że to z nią chciałem spędzić całe życie. Bez niej widzę tylko ciemność.

**Extract 24**

Kochałem ją nie mogłem znieść myśli że mnie odrzuciła

Życzę jej szczęścia

**Extract 25**

Przekaż [last_name] że go zawsze kochałam i nigdy o nim nie zapomnę. Najlepiej pokaż mu ten list. Bo to też przez niego się zajebałam. To był jedyny chłopak na którym mi tak zależało. Dla niego chciałam się zabić. Co właśnie pokazałam. Było mi zawsze tak dobrze jak z nim byłam... a on tylko sobie jaja robił. Trudno. [first name] już więcej na dyskotekę razem nie pójdziemy.

**Extract 26**

Witam wszystkich!!!
he he, mi jest do śmiechu a Wam nie? Nie zamulać!!!
Ja się zmieniam a tu kop od życia. Kurwa mać!!!
Wybaczcie mi...
Kocham Was wszystkich!!!
[first name]

**Extract 27**

Zabiłaś
Zabiłaś
Zabiłaś
Zabiłaś

**Extract 28**

Masz co chciałaś

**Extract 29**

Żegnaj już mnie nie będziesz dręczyć i bić zostawiam Ci wolną rękę

**Extract 30**

Byłam niedobrą żoną i matką. Ja tak dalej nie mogę żyć.

**Extract 31**

Sam tak niedawno mi powiedziałeś,że albo „łeb" mi ukręcisz, albo je wyrwiesz choćby nawet własnymi rękoma! Nigdy bym się tego po Tobie nie spodziewała bo uważałam Cię za wszystko co jest najpiękniejsze i najcudowniejsze!!! Ale Ty pokazałeś swoją drugą twarz, wyzywając mnie od najgorszych potworów, słuchałam tego i milczałam, bo nadal jesteś dla mnie „tym kochanym [person_name]" nadal, pomimo tych wszystkich słów! Pomimo tego, że uderzyłeś mnie wtedy w aucie! Było mi przykro, ale z każdym dniem próbowałam to jakoś sobie wytłumaczyć, ale już dłużej nie mogę, nie potrafię i nie chcę, chcę umrzeć i skrócić mój ból i cierpienie, które mi zadałeś...

**Extract 32**

zaczynam myśleć ym: o córce. że teraz (.) ona mi [głos jej się łamie] uświadomiła że m: (.) [cmoka] pokazała mi jak bardzo mnie kocha jak bardzo jej zależy na mnie i że moja śmierć bardzo ją skrzywdzi. strasznie ją zrani i powiedziała że nie wie czy temu ona sama podoła. czy pogodzi się z tą sytuacją czy (.) sama nie targnie się na swoje życie [...] i z tego co się okazało ona mnie bardzo kocha. ona nie wyrzuca mi tego że nie/że uważa że byłam najlepszą matką jaką mogłam być. (.)

**Extract 33**

ja się przekonałam że jednak tym dzieciom na mnie zależy. że ja naprawdę jestem im potrzebna. (.) bo: mimo wszystko że mają swoje rodziny czy (ja) to to jednak jednak (.) kochają mnie jak matkę bo ja/ nie nie powiedziały mi nigdy tego no bo (.) uważają że to jest normalne że ja wiem o tym że oni mnie kochają prawda? bo jestem matką i oni <u>muszą</u> mnie kochać.

**Extract 34**

dzieci mi okazały to że ja jestem/ i powiedziały prawda? że ja im jestem jeszcze potrzebna (.) że mam dla kogo żyć i bo mam ich mam męża mam wnuki które strasznie też kocham ale ja wtedy w tym w tym momencie wtedy nie myślałam o nikim tylko o samej sobie prawda?

**Extract 35**

pierwsze dni jak leżałam na obserwacji to myślałam po co mnie uratowali? a później jak już moje dzieci zaczęły do mnie dzwonić zaczęliśmy rozmawiać pisać ze sobą to dzięki dzieciom moim zrozumiałam że zrobiłam duży błąd. bo one mnie naprawdę potrzebują. [...] tak jakby mnie uświadomiło razem z dziećmi że (.) dzieci w tym momencie są najważniejsze i: tylko ich zraniłam.

**Extract 36**

dzieci mi okazały to że ja jestem/ i powiedziały prawda? że ja im jestem jeszcze potrzebna (.) że mam dla kogo żyć i bo mam ich mam męża mam wnuki które strasznie też kocham ale ja wtedy w tym w tym momencie wtedy nie myślałam o nikim tylko o samej sobie prawda?

# 9 Conclusions

## Introduction

This book has been founded on our continued astonishment about how little we know of the individual taking their life as well as their perspective on the act. We still know little about the lived experience of suicide, both before the event and after the attempt. How do people about to kill themselves see themselves in relation to what they do or did? What does it mean to them? What is the role of their close ones in the process?

We, therefore, positioned this book firmly as an examination of lived experience of suicide. We situated it in contrast to the dominant suicidological tradition. The goal was to see suicide through the eyes of those who are engaged in the process and we achieved it by exploring two sets of data: suicide notes and post-attempt interviews. What follows is the summary of the main points of the book.

### *The 'I' in Suicide*

Our first significant finding is the tension between institutional and lived representations of the self in relation to suicide. Institutional and activist discourses consistently remove the self and its agency from accounts of suicide. To them, suicides happen, and people die—as if it all just happened to them. References to people taking their lives are dealt with by sets of variables. Suicidology does not look at an individual person with their own narrated perspective on the world. Experience of suicide, whether narrated in suicide letters or post-attempt interviews, is largely unexplored in mainstream positivist suicidology. To a considerable extent, the top-down research perspective adopted by suicidology prevents suicidologists from exploring individual experiences.

One of the aims of this book was to offer a counter-perspective to such an approach to suicide. We adopted a bottom-up approach, focusing on

DOI: 10.4324/9781032672847-9

suicide through the lens of lived experience. As such, our research shows a significant difference between institutional and lived accounts of suicide. Stories of people engaged in suicidal processes show different relevancies to those in institutional discourses. There are two aspects of such differences.

First, while institutional discourses remove the individual from suicide while at the same time retaining its suicidal nature, lived accounts do the opposite. People writing suicide notes consistently stress their agency in taking their lives. They just do not readily call it suicide. The two kinds of discourses appear to be diametrically opposed, with relevancies that are in opposition to each other. Our research reveals that both institutional and activist discourses are detached from experience they either describe or advocate for. This makes them irrelevant to lived experience and, possibly, counter-productive and counter-useful.

The second finding we would like to highlight is that our explorations of agency in suicide offered new insights into the process of killing oneself. While agency in the stories of taking one's life is generally complex and fluctuating, it is agency behind waiting that was particularly surprising. People wanting to take their lives represent themselves as in full control of not ending their lives.

This finding is important because our research suggests a change of perspective in looking at suicide. We focus on a set of practices that at the time of crisis are responsible for life and survival. Our study is in agreement with Stritzke and Page (2020) who propose that suicidology should be more interested in asking the question of why people do not take their lives, despite suicidal ideation and wishes. By focusing on agency in waiting, we offer a largely ignored perspective in suicide research, exploring the entirety of the suicidal process, its dynamics, and also the pressure points possibly leading to protection and to death.

Our research suggests that it is crucial to focus on the experience of taking one's life, and, more importantly, on the experience of the process of not killing oneself. Waiting has been identified as protective at the macro level. In other words, people with suicidal ideation do not take their lives knowing that they have the means and could do it later (Brand et al., 2015). What our research shows is that such a strategy could also be seen at the local level of a single attempt. 'Wait some more' might well be protective here and now.

Our argument stems from our data in which the suicide process is constructed as calm and measured without drama or chaos. In such a way, the temptation to see waiting as indecision or ambivalence must be resisted. We propose that this is an important route for further research, and can lead to a deeper understanding of suicide and, crucially, new strategies in suicide prevention.

Our bottom-up perspective, at least in part, stems from the kinds of data we use. Suicide notes are very attractive for such research because they are unsolicited. The interviews, on the other hand, are a result of interactions with researchers whose aim is to offer their interviewees space for unrestrained narratives.

Moreover, farewell letters have different addressees and are likely to have different communicative goals. Unsolicited suicide notes allow ecological research and offer the possibility of a data-driven, bottom-up understanding of how suicide and everything around it are experienced by the person on the verge of taking their life. Suicide notes are texts preceding suicidal death and concomitant with the activities of suicide. In fact, they might be part of them. It is also worth pointing out that suicide notes are written, though the medium has been changing with the rise of digital notes (Ruder et al., 2011).

On the other hand, interviews with people who survived a suicide attempt offer a post-hoc perspective on what happened. We learn about suicide from people who attempted to kill themselves; they can tell us their stories in the interactional space we offer in the interviews.

The juxtaposition of accounts, underpinned by social scientific notions of triangulating data from such different datasets, has allowed us to see the suicide process from different points of view and offer a fuller picture of what it means to commit suicide. Moreover, the use of the two datasets with different representation interests (Kress & van Leeuwen, 1996) and communicative goals suggests the futility of reaching a 'true' account and the 'real' suicide. These stories offer a context-bound glimpse of suicide and not any semblance of the objective reality of suicide.

Indeed, suicidology's attempt to reach and describe a uniform act of suicide must be seen as unattainable. An understanding of how individuals experience suicidal thoughts and actions can facilitate a shift away from a biomedical model of suicide that often emphasises mental disorders. There is a need to focus on the existential and contextual factors that are of critical importance in suicidality (Hjelmeland & Knizek, 2017).

It is also worth stressing here that both suicide letters and interviews are primarily texts. We posit that discourse analysis is particularly well-suited for examining such texts. Indeed, we are astonished by the fact that there is still very little research that uses methods specifically aimed at analysing text, both in terms of its contents and, crucially, linguistic form (Testoni et al., 2021).

### *Suicide and its Meanings*

Suicide is commonly assumed to be the end of things. Whether it is assumed to bring the end of life or the end of consciousness, suicide is a person's final act. Our research contradicts such assumptions. Suicide must not be considered as universally ending things. Our data suggest that—at least in suicide notes—suicide can be positioned as a beginning.

We observed the view of suicide as a beginning, particularly in notes that romanticised suicide. In such notes, suicide was portrayed as leading to positive outcomes and, in some cases, affording the suicidal individual their '15 minutes of fame'. Suicide was represented as opening new channels of communication, informing people about the person and the act.

Suicide is positioned similarly in accounts of relationships. Assurances of love and care suggest that suicide does not end anything. In fact, in the suicide letters, individuals request continuing bonds from the addressees. The addressees can also be requested to continue with their feelings for the person who took their life.

It is worth adding that such findings tie in well with earlier analyses of suicide notes (Galasiński, 2017). We suggest that suicide notes construct suicide as if it did not end a person's life. Our analyses suggest that such representations are more common than might be expected. Both the person's agency and relationships are retained after the suicidal action.

Representations of suicide in suicide notes raise again the issue of their communicative status. In suicidological research, farewell letters are rarely problematised. Little has changed since the first ever study of suicide notes (Shneidman & Farberow, 1957); suicide notes are not considered acts of communication and are consistently positioned as offering insight into the suicidal mind. Suicide is seen as an event rather than a process underpinned by socially situated actions, while suicide notes are letters with content but without form or communicative function (for a more in-depth discussion on research into suicide notes, see Galasiński, 2017).

There are two points we would like to make here. First, suicide notes are not communicatively transparent; they are not a simple account of some realities, mostly underscored by the representational function.

**Extract 1**

You killed. You killed. You killed. You killed.

**Extract 2**

You have got what you wanted.

Such suicide notes as Extracts 1 and 2 can hardly be assumed as informing the addressees of anything. The information function of the text is at best secondary here, if important at all. Both notes are likely to be intended and received as blame, reproach, regret, or complaining. Indeed, the communicative functions of such notes are complex. Such complexity stems from particular relationships set up by the writers of the notes with the addressees.

Every interaction involves positioning the interactants with regard to each other (Davies & Harre, 1990). The blaming and reproaching recast such relationships to a moral or ethical dimension with the addressee becoming an accused, with all the cultural connotations it carries. In addition to this, such positioning must also be seen as self-presentational. Following Goffman's work (1959), such interactions involve 'facework', that is representation of oneself in a positive light. Becoming a victim at least has the potential of positioning the deceased favourably. The two notes therefore can hardly be seen as simply offering insight into the mind of the authors. Rather, they are likely to be intended to bear a social and psychological impact on those who would read them. In other words, being blamed so directly is likely not only to be read and understood, but also to evoke a reaction in both the immediate addressees and those around them.

Authors of suicide letters confessed love, accused, apologised, thanked, promised, and asked for forgiveness. In all such notes, different relationships are set up, different self-images are invoked, and crucially, different points are scored. Consider also the following extract:

**Extract 3**

I will haunt you and [name] till you are alive.

The note is likely intended to be a threat to the addressee. Assuming that the writer is a competent user of language, they must have realised that this is how the note is likely to be understood. Not only can the note not (and ought not to) be interpreted as a direct reflection of the author's thoughts, but it also constructs a relationship with an assumed power dynamic between the author and the addressee. The power it is worth stressing, he will wield from the beyond the grave.

While the representational value of the note is fairly straightforward, its communicative functions are less so. Any analysis must begin with the question of whether the note should be taken at face value, while any decision might or might not coincide with how the note will be interpreted by the addressee. To make matters more complex, there are bound to be contexts to which such analyses cannot speak. For example, did the note author believe in spiritual life? Does the note refer to some private event, perhaps even a joke? There are so many permutations of (inter-)subjectivities used in writing and understanding the notes that such questions could go on indefinitely. And while the analysis based on the linguistic form is sound, it might not be full at all.

Such considerations raise one last issue we would like to raise here. By positioning suicide letters as a gateway to the author's mind, suicidological research tacitly assumes that such texts are honest and sincere acts of communication. In other words, those writing suicide letters simply 'speak their minds'. There is no reason to assume that at all. Indeed, controversial as such points might be, we do not doubt that suicide notes can be written strategically, perhaps also manipulatively. It is important to stress that there is no reason to assume that normal rules of communication, be it social, cultural, or psychological, stop working.

Considering our earlier points about suicide not ending relationships, the note in Extract 3 might well be considered a manipulative attempt to interfere with another existing relationship with the note author's partner. Indeed, there are several notes in which men quite explicitly talk about making sure that their partners/wives must not engage in relationships or sex with other men.

A suicide note might well be the last opportunity to score one, take revenge, or get your own back. There is no reason to assume that just because a person wants to take their life, all ulterior motives disappear. Given the number of notes confessing eternal love and stressing the inability to live without the person left behind, it seems there is at least a significant context for messages with complex social and psychological goals underpinning them. And so, to reiterate, suicide notes must not be seen as transparent texts simply rendering what the note authors thought or felt. If anything, they should be treated as the exact opposite of that. Suicide notes are sites of complex, multipurpose acts of communication, possibly with hidden, strategic, or manipulative goals both for the self and those around it.

### *Suicide is Entangled*

The final theme we explore in the book can be subsumed by a statement that suicide is entangled. We argue that suicide must not be assumed to be an individual act. Time and again, both in the suicide letters and in the interviews, suicides were positioned in relation to others. This was done in two ways.

First, we examined stories of suicidal parents. The picture painted by parents' suicide letters is mixed. On the one hand, both fathers and mothers address and describe their children in positive ways, while, on the other, children are accused of hurting their parents. Suicide was constructed as having an aftermath. Parents consistently wanted to leave a legacy behind.

In such stories, suicide became a means to endow children with gifts; alternatively, suicide was the beginning of future love and care.

The second aspect of suicide entanglement is its relationship with love. Suicide cannot override the love a person feels, which is their bequest for the future. Alternatively, love can be destructive and even though suicide is rarely blamed on the loved one, love is a source of misery. Yet, love is also protective. Stories of those who survived their suicide attempts talked about the love of those around them. It is such love that is described as having the power to save a person from future suicide attempts.

In making such points, we are mindful of the fact that suicidology is largely uninterested in these contexts and the roles people play in a suicidal individual's life. While much literature explores family-related risk factors, there is little suicidological interest in the relationship contexts and experiences in individual suicides. Such literature rarely goes beyond seeing relationships as variables to be measured. Connectedness is viewed as part of the behavioural and motivational moderators rather than as a context-dependent and dynamic set of experiences. What we see as a complex experience of a person with their context-dependent subjectivities and identities, always in a dynamic relationship with others, is largely unexplored in suicidological research. In such a scenario, suicide cannot be seen as a new meaningful context in which relationships are re-negotiated, also, paradoxically, after suicidal death.

In our view, such arguments are important for how suicidological research is carried out. Suicide must be positioned as a context-bound process constituted by individuals' experiences and actions. It is in stark contrast with the view of suicide as a dot on a timeline, or a singular event in which individual participation is seen in terms of sets of variables. The result from it is research focusing primarily on correlates of suicide, especially those that can be described as risk factors; second, it is warning signs of suicide. Discoveries of new risk factors are greeted with postulates that more should be examined. This is the way, it is argued, successful intervention and prevention strategies can be developed (British Psychological Society [BPS], 2017). In such a research agenda, suicide itself remains largely unexplored.

Indeed, we tend to be sceptical of the multiple models and theories of suicide, such as Interpersonal Theory of Suicide (Joiner, 2005; Van Orden, Witte, Cukrowicz, Braithwaite, Selby, & Joiner, 2010), Reciprocity-Based Theory (Davis et al., 2009), and existential-constructivist model of suicide (Rogers, 2001), to name just a few (Gunn & Lester, 2014). To our knowledge, these models do not offer much in terms of the explanatory power of suicide as a context-bound and embodied series of actions.

We posit that qualitative research offers a way forward for suicidology, and, indeed, our previous work is a good example of the usefulness of such research (e.g., Galasiński, 2017; Galasiński & Ziółkowska, 2020). The most significant advantage of such research is that it allows researchers to focus on the act of suicide as it is experienced by those engaged in it. We realise, of course, also in qualitative research, that access to suicide itself is necessarily indirect. Neither the *ex-ante* (suicide notes) nor the *post-hoc* (interviews) accounts offer anything that could be seen as the 'truth'. Qualitative research is capable only of studying stories or accounts that construct the events of which they speak. As ever, they are subject to the usual social and psychological pressures, just as in the case of communication in any setting. Still, the qualitative perspective offers the possibility of focusing on the very centre of suicidological concern. We believe that without understanding suicide and its meanings, effective preventive or therapeutic actions are significantly hampered, if they make sense at all (Hjelmeland, 2010; Leenaars, 2002; Hjelmeland & Knizek, 2010; 2017).

### *Suicide Prevention*

At the moment, psychological strategies in suicide prevention are based on top-down theoretical models with practically no reference to what is known about the experience of suicide or suicide attempts, be it through suicide notes or *post hoc* interviews (McCabe et al., 2018). The primary focus is on risk factors.

Identification of risk factors associated with suicidal thoughts and behaviours is often considered crucial in the development of effective prevention strategies. Risk factors are thought to identify individuals at increased risk of suicide, even though it is also accepted that they are poor and imprecise predictors of suicidal behaviour. Franklin et al. (2017) demonstrated that there has been no improvement in predictive ability over the previous 50 years of research. In a nutshell, instruments used for assessing suicide risk do not work. Their positive predictive power is as little as 5% (Carter et al., 2017; see also: Belsher et al., 2019). This is not a good result by any stretch of the imagination. Incidentally, despite this, and the fact that clinical guidelines (especially in the United Kingdom) recommend that such assessments not be used, they continue to be (Quinlivan et al., 2014).

This is particularly significant in light of research indicating multiple pathways in the suicidal process, including the progression to suicidal behaviour without prior suicidal thoughts or a premeditated plan. A substantial body of research indicates that a considerable proportion of individuals who engage in suicidal behaviour may not acknowledge the presence of suicidal ideation and/or premeditated planning (Bryan et al., 2023). Such patients do not report suicidal thoughts and plans, so tools used to assess suicide may result in missed opportunities to intervene with people who may be at high risk, but do not have overt suicidal ideation.

This is indeed why we agree with the perspective on suicide prevention taken by Kapur and Goldney (2019). The basic tenet of their approach is to focus on the individual needs of a patient. Suicide prevention means providing good quality individualised healthcare in which the patient is treated as a partner rather than an object of medical action.

Personal narratives can be seen as a proxy for lived experience that offer both the researcher and the clinician the possibility of focusing on the individual and their experiences, and through this, their individual needs. Our approach also acknowledges that risk is dynamic and context-bound and that the individual is in control of their behaviour (action) and desires. Indeed, we understand that stories of suicide are subject to social constraints such as stigma, which can result in some self-censorship among individuals who are thinking about it. Feeling ashamed or embarrassed about suicidal thoughts may prevent suicidal people from talking openly about their thoughts during clinical assessment (DeVylder et al., 2022). The clinician's prejudices or misconceptions about suicide may also serve to alienate the suicidal person.

Now, the results of our research raise two other points. First, if suicide is understood as a set of actions taken by a socially entangled individual and not a single act, this must have consequences for risk assessment, and therefore, suicide prevention. It is unlikely that there is a uniform set of 'suicide prevention' actions for everyone. Instead, prevention strategies must consider the fact that suicide is not a one-off, homogeneous act that can be prevented; it stems from the socially situated experiences of individuals. It is research exploration of such experiences that is paramount to understanding suicide and planning prevention strategies. We are aware, of course, that this complicates prevention strategies significantly, and we are also aware that our proposal might well mean shifting prevention strategies from the macro-level of the society onto the micro-level of the individual stories.

Both suicide prevention and risk assessment and management should be done with the individual. Approaches of collaboration in the assessment and management of suicide risk already exist, most notably as the Collaborative Assessment and Management of Suicidality (CAMS) developed by Jobes and co-authors (2016). We think that a deeper understanding of individual narratives afforded by discourse analysis will enhance our understanding of risk, meaning, and experience of suicide.

We also propose that discourse analysis can be useful in planning and designing suicide prevention strategies. It facilitates the acquisition of insights into the lived experiences of individuals with suicidal thoughts, or history of suicidal behaviours. Discourse analysis and qualitative methodologies encourage analytical efforts and insights from diverse lived experiences thereby informing prevention and intervention strategies and procedures. It is only through such approaches that researchers and prevention strategists can learn about the complexities of suicidal behaviour (Espeland et al., 2021; Hjelmeland & Knizek, 2010; Bantjes & Swartz, 2019). This is of particular importance in light of the necessity of tailoring suicide prevention, and intervention strategies and practices, to specific populations at risk (Kabir et al., 2023).

As discourse analysis allows examining first-person accounts of suicide experience, it can offer insight both into patterns of such experience and the relevancies underpinning it. When combined with ethnographic observation (Hammersley & Atkinson, 2019), it can offer a triangulated view of the lived experience of suicide. Such analyses can also place the experiences in the context of power dynamics surrounding suicide, thereby resulting in a fuller discovery and understanding of social meanings that shape individual and collective experiences related to suicide. Indeed, examining how discourses about suicide contribute to the perpetuation of stigma and shape the experiences of individuals who attempted suicide or those who experienced the loss of a loved one to suicide (Pitman et al., 2018) seems an obvious way forward.

Given the diverse subject positions that individuals occupy in everyday life, it is unsurprising that their attitudes towards suicide can also be complex and contradictory. Discourse analysis can assist in identifying the various competing narratives surrounding suicide. A notable example is the study conducted by Conrad and Coohey (2023), which employed a contrapuntal analysis to discern meanings among online suicide chat users. Their findings revealed the emergence of two distinct discourses, namely Discourses of the Precious Life (DPL) and Discourses of Life as a Thing (DLT), which competed with each other in their attempts to make meaning of suicide.

In summary, we think that the results of our qualitative discourse analysis offer at least two new perspectives on suicide prevention. On the one hand, it is understanding suicide as a more complex set of events and developing strategies to deal with them. On the other hand, we think that suicide prevention should stem from individuals' experiences and be focused more on individuals' needs underpinned by insight from individual narrated experiences. Finally, we would like to stress that what we suggested above is not a suggestion of revolution. Rather, it is viewing current calls for change in suicidology and in suicide prevention given our research as well as the assumptions underpinning qualitative research with discourse analytic focus.

## We Want to be Useful

Ultimately, this book aims to be useful. Our most basic argument is that accounts of suicide offer a lived perspective on how an individual experiences suicide in the complex contexts they find themselves. Through such stories, we can see the individual as they are narrated, without reducing them to a set of variables. Such accounts are in some conflict with how suicidology understands and explores suicide. We think that it is the unique perspectives of individual stories that are more useful in how we, as researchers, should understand suicide and its experience. It is the lived experience that offers a deeper understanding of how suicide is experienced and makes sense of both the beginning and the end of the process.

Our final contention is that text-based studies are particularly interesting when trying to tease out the discourses of people with experiences of suicide. It is the lexico-grammatical form of how people speak or write that allows researchers and clinicians solid evidence not only of social practices and beliefs around suicide but also a solid base of clinical practice. In other words, it is an insight into the working of the narrative that can be the basis of clinical assessment as both representatives of narrative medicine and narrative psychology would argue (Greenhalgh & Hurwitz, 1998; Charon & Wyer, 2008; Brockmeier & Carbaugh, 2001). And so we argue that text-based discourse analysis can be a significant resource not merely for research into suicide and its distress but also clinical and preventative practice. Discourse analysis can be a powerful toolkit helping the practitioner (whether engaged in clinical action or suicide prevention) in unpicking the experiences of those who are at their most vulnerable. This unpicking, which we have shown throughout this book, can lead to more nuanced and hence better strategies to understand suicide.

Suicide takes us to the edge of experience. Beyond it, the experience ends. Perhaps this metaphor of suicide as a precipice that takes us where we are no longer, offered a context in which suicide is seen as an act without structure and outside time. In such a perspective, suicide becomes only a step off the precipice. We call for a view of suicide that acknowledges both the experience and subjectivities involved in it. We also argue for acknowledging that people do not just jump off the edge. There is much to be done before they do that. We think that understanding it will not only help us understand those people and their experiences but also lead to helping them better.

## References

Bantjes, J., & Swartz, L. (2019). 'What can we learn from first-person narratives?' The case of nonfatal suicidal behavior. *Qualitative Health Research*, *29*(10), 1497–1507. https://doi.org/10.1177/1049732319832869

Belsher, B., Smolenski, D., Pruitt, L., Bush, N., Beech, E., Workman, D., Morgan, R. L., Evatt, D. P., Tucker, J., & Skopp, N. (2019). Prediction models for suicide attempts and deaths. *JAMA Psychiatry*, *76*(6), 642–651. https://doi.org/10.1001/jamapsychiatry.2019.0174

British Psychological Society [BPS]. (2017). *Position statement. Understanding and preventing suicide: A psychological perspective.* Retrieved from: https://pure.strath.ac.uk/ws/portalfiles/portal/153526698/Arensman_etal_TP_2017_Position_statement_understanding_and_preventing_suicide.pdf

Brand, S. L., Gibson, S., & Benson, O. (2015). Planning on dying to live: A qualitative exploration of the alleviation of suicidal distress by having a suicide plan. *Suicidology Online*, *6*(2), 61–68.

Brockmeier, J., & Carbaugh, D. (Eds.). (2001). *Narrative and identity: Studies in autobiography, self and culture.* John Benjamins Publishing Company. https://doi.org/10.1075/sin.1

Bryan, C. J., Allen, M. H., Wastler, H. M., Bryan, A. O., Baker, J. C., May, A. M., & Thomsen, C. J. (2023). Rapid intensification of suicide risk preceding suicidal behavior among primary care patients. *Suicide and Life-Threatening Behavior*, *53*(3), 352–361. https://doi.org/10.1111/sltb.12948

Carter, G., Milner, A., McGill, K., Pirkis, J., Kapur, N., & Spittal, M. J. (2017). Predicting suicidal behaviours using clinical instruments: Systematic review and meta-analysis of positive predictive values for risk scales. *British Journal of Psychiatry*, *210*(6), 387–395. https://doi.org/10.1192/bjp.bp.116.182717

Charon, R., & Wyer, P. (2008). Narrative evidence-based medicine. *The Lancet*, *371*(9609), 296–297. https://doi.org/10.1016/s0140-6736(08)60156-7

Conrad, J. B., & Coohey, C. (2023). The constructed meaning of suicide: A relational dialectics theory analysis of online suicide chats. *Journal of Communication Inquiry*, *47*(2), 168–186. https://doi.org/10.1177/01968599221128533

Davies, B., & Harré, R. (1990). Positioning: The discursive production of selves. *Journal for the Theory of Social Behaviour*, *20*(1), 43–63. https://doi.org/10.1111/j.1468-5914.1990.tb00174.x

Davis, M. S., Callanan, V. J., Lester, D., & Haines, J. (2009). An inquiry into relationship suicides and reciprocity. *Suicide and Life-Threatening Behavior*, *39*(5), 482–498. https://doi.org/10.1521/suli.2009.39.5.482

DeVylder, J., Yang, L., Goldstein, R., Ross, A., Oh, H., Zhou, S., Horowitz, L., & Bridge, J. (2022). Mental health correlates of stigma among college students with suicidal ideation: Data from the 2020–2021 healthy minds study. *Stigma and Health*, *7*(2), 247–250. https://doi.org/10.1037/sah0000376

Espeland, K., Knizek, B., & Hjelmeland, H. (2021). 'Time to try something new'—professionals' experiences and reflections on suicide prevention in Norway. *Crisis*, *42*(6), 434–440. https://doi.org/10.1027/0227-5910/a000740

Franklin, J. C., Ribeiro, J. D., Fox, K. R., Bentley, K. H., Kleiman, E. M., Huang, X., ... & Nock, M. K. (2017). Risk factors for suicidal thoughts and behaviors: A meta-analysis of 50 years of research. *Psychological Bulletin*, *143*(2), 187–232. https://doi.org/10.1037/bul0000084

Galasiński, D. (2017). *Discourses of men's suicide notes: A qualitative analysis.* Bloomsbury.

Galasiński, D., & Ziółkowska, J. (2020). *Discursive constructions of the suicidal process.* Bloomsbury.

Goffman, E. (1959). *The presentation of self in everyday life*, Garden City: Doubleday.

Greenhalgh, T., & Hurwitz, B. (1999). Why study narrative? *BMJ*, *318*(7175), 48–50. https://doi.org/10.1136/bmj.318.7175.48
Gunn, J. F., & Lester, D. (2014). *Theories of suicide: Past, present and future*. Charles C Thomas Publisher.
Hammersley, M., & Atkinson, P. (2019). *Ethnography. Principles in practice* (4th ed.). Routledge.
Hjelmeland, H. (2010). Cultural research in suicidology: Challenges and opportunities. *Suicidology Online*, *1*(1), 34–52.
Hjelmeland, H., & Knizek, B. L. (2010). Why we need qualitative research in suicidology. *Suicide and Life-Threatening Behavior*, *40*(1), 74–80. https://doi.org/10.1521/suli.2010.40.1.74
Hjelmeland, H., & Knizek, B. L. (2017). Suicide and mental disorders: A discourse of politics, power, and vested interests. *Death Studies*, *41*(8), 481–492. https://doi.org/10.1080/07481187.2017.1332905
Jobes, D. A., Comtois, K. A., Brenner, L. A., Gutierrez, P. M., & O'Connor, S. S. (2016). Lessons learned from clinical trials of the Collaborative Assessment and Management of Suicidality (CAMS). In Rory C. O'Connor & Jane Pirkis (Eds.), *The international handbook of suicide prevention* (pp. 431–449). John Wiley & Sons, Ltd. https://doi.org/10.1002/9781118903223.ch24
Joiner, Jr, T. E. (2005). *Why people die by suicide*. Harvard University Press.
Kabir, H., Wayland, S. & Maple, M. (2023). Qualitative research in suicidology: A systematic review of the literature of low-and middle-income countries. *BMC Public Health* 23(1), 918. https://doi.org/10.1186/s12889-023-15767-9
Kapur, N., & Goldney, R. D. (2019). *Suicide prevention*. Oxford University Press.
Kress, G., & van Leeuwen, T. (1996). *Reading images*. Routledge.
Leenaars, A. A. (2002). The quantitative and qualitative in suicidological science: An editorial. *Archives of Suicide Research*, *6*(1), 1–3. https://doi.org/10.1080/13811110213121
McCabe, R., Garside, R., Backhouse, A., & Xanthopoulou, P. (2018). Effectiveness of brief psychological interventions for suicidal presentations: A systematic review. *BMC Psychiatry*, *18*, 1–13. https://doi.org/10.1186/s12888-018-1663-5
Pitman, A., Stevenson, F., Osborn, D., & King, M. (2018). The stigma associated with bereavement by suicide and other sudden deaths: A qualitative interview study. *Social Science & Medicine*, *198*, 121–129. https://doi.org/10.1016/j.socscimed.2017.12.035
Quinlivan, L., Cooper, J., Steeg, S., Davies, L., Hawton, K., Gunnell, D., & Kapur, N. (2014). Scales for predicting risk following self-harm: An observational study in 32 hospitals in England. *BMJ Open*, *4*(5), e004732. https://doi.org/10.1136/bmjopen-2013-004732
Rogers, J. R. (2001). Theoretical grounding: The 'missing link' in suicide research. *Journal of Counseling & Development*, *79*(1), 16–25. https://doi.org/10.1002/j.1556-6676.2001.tb01939.x
Ruder, T. D., Hatch, G. M., Ampanozi, G., Thali, M. J., & Fischer, N. (2011). Suicide announcement on Facebook. *Crisis*, *32*(5), 280–282. https://doi.org/10.1027/0227-5910/a000086

Shneidman, E. S., & Farberow, N. L. (1957). Some comparisons between genuine and simulated suicide notes in terms of Mowrer's concepts of discomfort and relief. *The Journal of General Psychology*, *56*(2), 251–256.

Stritzke, W. G. K., & Page, A. C. (2020). Suicide is about life. In A. C. Page & W. G. K. Stritzke (Eds.), *Alternatives to suicide. Beyond risk and toward a life worth living* (pp. 89–110). Academic Press.

Testoni, I., De Vincenzo, C., & Zamperini, A. (2021). The words to say it—Qualitative suicide research. In K. Kõlves, M. Sisask, P. Värnik, A. Värnik & D. De Leo (Eds.), *Advancing suicide research* (pp. 129–150). Hogrefe.

Van Orden, K. A., Witte, T. K., Cukrowicz, K. C., Braithwaite, S. R., Selby, E. A., & Joiner Jr, T. E. (2010). The interpersonal theory of suicide. *Psychological Review*, *117*(2), 575–600.

## Appendix

### Extract 1

Zabiłaś
Zabiłaś
Zabiłaś
Zabiłaś

### Extract 2

Masz co chciałaś

### Extract 3

I ciebie i oraz [name] będę straszył dokąd będziecie żyli

# Index


action 2–3, 6, 8–9, 13–14, 16–18, 25–6, 38, 41–7, 49, 51–4, 63–4, 66–7, 69–70, 72–8, 86–8, 94, 109, 111, 114, 117–21, 132–3, 137, 153, 159, 176, 179, 201, 204–8
aftermath 2, 162, 172, 203
agency 2–3, 8–13, 17–19, 24–5, 38–41, 43–4, 46–54, 63–77, 86, 117–19, 121, 174, 177, 198–9, 201; loss of agency 9–10, 44, 47–9
ambivalence 10, 49, 69, 71–4, 76–7, 96, 112, 119, 135, 153, 160, 182, 199; research 76
American Psychiatric Association (APA) 5, 13, 39–41, 43, 173
ancient Greece 5, 10
apologies 98, 112–14, 121
assumptions 15–16, 48, 54, 109, 141, 200–1, 207

belongingness 9, 188–9 *see also* thwarted belongingness/love
bereavement 5, 10, 95, 132, 152–3
biomedical model 6, 200 *see also* medicalisation
bottom-up perspectives 2, 16, 19, 77, 198–200
bravery 24, 48, 87, 162
Broz, Ludek 8, 64
burdensome 9, 111
burial 11–12, 93–4

celebration 89, 91–2, 99
celebrities 87–8, 99–100
childhood 135–7, 142, 151
classification systems 6, 39–40, 173
coffins 9, 94
conceptual models/frameworks 10, 39–40, 42
confessions 112–15, 133, 135–8, 140–1, 160, 175, 177, 179–80, 183, 188
conflict 13, 110, 131, 152–3, 173, 199, 208
connectedness 110, 111, 130, 188–9, 204
control 3, 5, 8–9, 12, 24, 68–78, 119, 199, 206
coping 10, 52, 69, 112, 140, 184
copycat suicidal behaviour *see* Werther effect
counterbalance 67, 160
crime 5, 10–11, 24
Critical Discourse Analysis (CDA) 13–16, 18–19 *see also* discourse analysis

data/dataset 14–15, 21–4, 73, 76–8, 88–9, 109, 111, 119–21, 128–9, 131–2, 135–6, 139–40, 142, 151, 158, 182, 184–5, 187, 189, 198, 200–1
definitions 6–7, 12, 44–7
depart/ leave 51, 97, 111, 117, 133, 136–7, 159–61, 163, 188, 203
*Diagnostic and Statistical Manual of Mental Disorders* (DSM) 5, 19, 39–43, 47–8, 173
diagnostic manuals 39–40, 44–5, 53
directives 88–9, 91, 93, 96, 99, 178
discourse analysis 1–2, 4, 21, 77, 200, 206–8 *see also* Critical Discourse Analysis (CDA)

discourses: institutional 25, 38, 47, 49–50, 53–4, 63, 199; public 38, 47, 49–50, 53, 88, 109
distress 12, 40, 151, 172–3, 208
dominant models/paradigms 1, 3, 8, 10, 20, 25, 39, 43, 46, 77, 120, 141, 154, 161, 163, 174, 198
drama 1, 3, 23, 73, 77, 97–9, 101, 164, 179, 199

ethics approval 21–2
ethnography 9–10, 207
euphemism 50–1, 53, 113

farewells 26, 51, 92, 96–7, 101, 109, 113–14, 139, 164, 172, 179, 182, 200–1
fatherhood 129, 154–5, 161–3 *see also* parenthood
forgiveness 50–1, 69, 90, 98, 112–15, 131–4, 154, 157, 159, 176, 182, 202
funerals 88, 90–4, 99, 101

gender 3–4, 8, 23, 129, 152–3
gifts 95, 115–16, 121, 153–6, 161, 164, 183–4, 204
guilt 7, 78, 139–40, 174

Halliday, Michael 17–18, 131, 188
heroism 86–7
honour 5, 10, 87, 91
hopelessness 7, 9, 11, 111, 173, 187

ideology 15–16, 18, 129, 188
identities 18–19, 22–3, 109, 121, 158, 162–3, 204
illness 5, 10–11, 15, 18–20, 22, 39–40, 49, 51, 64, 87, 162, 173
informants 22–3, 26, 54, 69–71, 73, 118–21, 184, 186, 189 *see also* participants
intention 6, 8–9, 16, 38–9, 41, 44–5, 49, 64–5, 73–4
*International Classification of Mental and Behavioural Disorders* (ICD) 19, 39–40, 44, 46
Interpersonal Theory of Suicide (IPTS) 9, 20, 111, 130, 204
intervention strategies 4, 10, 42, 88, 204, 206–7
interviews 3, 8–9, 14–15, 21–3, 26, 49, 51–3, 70–1, 73–6, 101, 109, 111, 117–18, 120–1, 128, 153, 184, 187–90, 198, 200, 203, 205
isolation 22, 110–11

juxtaposition 25, 47, 49, 63, 67, 75, 137, 139–40, 162, 176, 200

leave *see* depart/leave
legacy 2, 26, 142, 151–7, 161–4, 172, 188, 203–4
letters 1, 23, 25–6, 51–2, 65–9, 71, 75–6, 88–92, 96–9, 109, 112–14, 116, 120–1, 128–9, 131–2, 135, 139, 141–2, 151–3, 155–62, 164, 175–84, 186–8, 198, 200–3
language 14–19, 23–4, 40, 42, 48–9, 77, 139, 182, 202 *see also* linguistics, Polish language
lexicogrammatical form 8, 16, 65, 208
life advice 26, 156–8
linguistics 13–17, 46–7, 51–2, 65, 77, 93, 116, 131, 139, 141, 157–60, 162–3, 174–5, 177–9, 182–3, 185, 188–9, 200, 203 *see also* language
lived experience 8, 10, 25, 38, 47, 49–54, 63, 88, 101, 121, 198–9, 206–8
love 4, 26, 48, 50, 66, 78, 87, 97, 112–15, 118, 132–40, 151, 153, 155–6, 159–64, 172–89, 201–4; destructive 178–9, 183–4, 187; eternal 114, 175, 183, 203; heartbreak 87, 173; stories 172–89 *see also* reciprocity

manipulation 8, 203
marginalisation 13, 19, 25, 40, 54, 63, 65, 67, 77, 86
margins of suicide 54, 63, 67, 77
Marsh, Ian 11–12, 15, 21, 64
media coverage 86–8, 99, 101, 187
mental processes 17, 42, 53, 131–2
medicalisation 5–6, 12–13, 15, 19, 39–40, 64 *see also* biomedical model
methodology 16–21, 76–7, 200, 206
moral obligation/perspective 49, 89, 129, 202
motherhood 130, 161, 163–4 *see also* parenthood
Münster, Daniel 8, 64

objects 8, 42, 44, 92
observation 87, 95, 207

pain 9, 54, 78, 87, 111–12, 133, 155, 183, 187–8
parenthood 26, 89, 120, 128–42, 151–64, 172–3, 203–4 *see also* fatherhood, motherhood
participants 7, 9, 17–18, 21–2, 48 *see also* informants
participation 46, 53, 129, 204
Polish language 22–4, 40, 43, 182
power 16, 18, 139, 154, 174, 188, 202, 204–5, 207–8
preparatory acts 41–2
psychiatry 5, 12–13, 15, 39–40, 42–4, 53, 64
punishment 10–12

qualitative research/process 2–4, 16, 19–22, 77, 173, 204–7
quantitative paradigm 8, 19–20, 163
questionnaires 9, 189

reciprocity 4, 26, 115, 177–9, 181, 183, 187–8
regret 26, 52, 116–20, 132, 202
rejection 3–4, 54, 70, 87, 118, 180–1, 187
relationships 2, 7, 9, 25–5, 51, 94, 96, 101, 110–12, 116–17, 120–1, 128, 131–2, 134, 137–8, 141, 151, 173–4, 178, 184, 186, 189, 201–4
remembrance 88, 177–8
representation 13–15, 17, 19, 25, 53–4, 69, 88, 100–1, 109, 112, 135, 137, 173, 187, 189, 198, 200–2
resolution 157, 173
responsibility 9–10, 50–1, 53, 63–4, 66, 112, 117, 119, 129–30, 153, 159, 178, 182

semiotics 13–16, 153
sensationalism 86–8
shame 7, 78, 87, 115, 138, 161, 163, 173, 206
Shneidman, Edwin S. 1, 7–9, 47, 76–8, 172, 174
social context 1–2, 7, 15, 17, 20, 40, 87
social practice 14–15, 185, 208
special events 92, 94
stigmatisation 22, 48–9, 52–4, 206–7
stories 1–4, 8, 22–3, 25, 38, 50, 63, 65, 71, 73, 78, 86–8, 109, 111, 118–20, 142, 151, 153, 164, 172, 177–8, 184, 187, 189, 199–200, 203–6, 208
suffering 1, 3–4, 7, 9, 132–3, 155, 183
suicidal behaviour disorder 5, 41, 173
suicide attempt 1–4, 6–7, 12, 15, 21, 23–4, 26, 39, 41–4, 50, 52–4, 63–5, 69, 71, 74–6, 110, 118, 121, 131, 164, 172–3, 184, 200, 204–5
suicide: dilemma 16, 109, 120, 188; experiences 3, 152, 207; notes 3–4, 8, 15, 21, 23, 26, 49–50, 53, 63, 66–7, 78, 88–9, 92, 96–101, 109, 111–12, 114–16, 120–1, 128, 135, 137, 140–1, 151–3, 156, 161, 172, 174–6, 184, 187–8, 198–203, 205; prevention 1–2, 4–6, 63, 100, 109, 120–1, 187, 199, 205–8; process 15, 68–9, 78, 86, 111, 117, 120–1, 187–8, 199–200
suicidology 1–4, 7–8, 12, 19–21, 45–7, 64, 77–8, 88–9, 99, 120, 141–2, 187, 198–200, 204–5, 207–8

text-based/oriented approach 3, 14, 19, 100, 208
theoretical perspectives 8, 121, 205
Three-Step Theory (3ST) 111
thwarted belongingness/love 7, 9, 109–11, 130, 179, 187–9 *see also* belongingness
tolerance 5, 10–11, 78
top-down perspectives 2, 77, 198, 205
tragedy 1, 24, 49, 100–1, 183
transitivity 17–18
translations 23–4, 40, 43

vocabulary 24–5
vulnerability 10, 87, 99–100, 111, 152, 208

waiting 25, 54, 63, 65–73, 76, 78, 86, 121, 199; active waiting 67
well-being 9, 128, 151
Werther effect 86–8, 99–100
World Health Organisation (WHO) 4–5, 39
writing 23, 26, 50, 67–8, 88, 96–100, 117–18, 128–9, 131–40, 151, 153, 157, 160–2, 164, 178, 185, 199, 202–3

For Product Safety Concerns and Information please contact our
EU representative GPSR@taylorandfrancis.com Taylor & Francis
Verlag GmbH, Kaufingerstraße 24, 80331 München, Germany